THE PILATES
EXERCISE ENCYCLOPEDIA

Vicky Timón

Publishing Director:
Juliana Esperança

Illustrations by:
Isabel Arechabala

Design and Layout:
Alberto Palomares

Translated by:
Sandra Elena Dermark

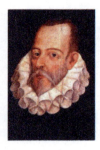 They call me Miguel de Cervantes Saavedra, and in 1605 I had printed a small volume which earned me great fame but little fortune.

The first year saw the fruit of my wit blown up into five editions, each as false as thieves, which caused no small hurt to my honor and no less loss to my scant estate.

In those days, there was no copyright as there is today.

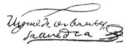

Moral: Please don't make pirate copies.
3rd edition, expanded and improved

© Pila Teleña, 2022
C/ Pozo Nuevo, 12
28430 Alpedrete, Madrid (Spain)
Telf: 609 25 20 82
editorial@pilatelena.com
www.pilatelena.com

ISBN: 978-84-16740-24-6
Legal Deposit: M-15768-2022
Made in the EU

All rights reserved. No part of this work may be reproduced or transmitted by any mechanical or digital means, including reprographic printing, without the prior permission in writing of the copyright holders. Within the meaning of this notice, reproduction and transmission include, inter alia, reprographic printing, digitization and the public rental or loan of copies, which is strictly prohibited without the prior consent of the publisher.

Respect copyright! A lot of people have put a lot of work into this book and they deserve their reward.

THE PILATES
EXERCISE ENCYCLOPEDIA

Vicky Timón

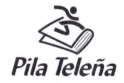

Pila Teleña

CONTENTS

Prolog 11
How to Use This Book 13
Introducing the Pilates Method 19

1. Exercises by Category 22

Basic Principles 23

   01. Cranio-Vertebral Articulation 26
   02. Scapular Stabilization 28
   03. Pelvic Stabilization 30
   04. Axial Elongation 34
   05. Abdominal Connection 36
   06. Body Alignment and Balance 38
   07. Breathing 40
   08. Integration and Control 44

Abdominal

   01. Ab Prep (1-1) 47
   02. Hundred (3-1) 50

03. Half Roll Back (4-1) 53
04. Roll Up (5-1) 56
05. Rolling Like a Ball (8-1) 58
06. One Leg Stretch (9-1) 60
07. One Leg Stretch Oblique (10-1) 62
08. Double Leg Stretch (11-1) 64
09. Scissors (12-1) 67
10. Half Roll Back Obliques (15-1) 69
11. Axial Flex (19-1) 72
12. Seal (21-1) 74
13. Trunk Rotation (24-1) 76
14. Abdominal Series (26-1) 78
15. Slow Double Leg Strech) (1-2) 81
16. Roll Over (3-2) 84
17. Open Leg Rocker (5-2) 86
18. Roll Up Advanced (6-2) 88
19. Teaser (Teaser) (9-2) 93
20. Hip Twist (12-2) 96
21. Teaser Series (2-3) 98
22. Teaser Series (2-3) 99
23. Corkscrew (6-3) 100
24. Boomerang (9-3) 102

Mixed

01. Twist (7-1) 105
02. Saw (14-1) 107
03. Trunk and Legs Lateral Elevation (18-1) 110

04. Cat And Horse (23-1) 111

05. Supine Squad (25-1) 114

06. Double Leg Kick (8-2) 116

07. Swimming (10-2) 119

08. Leg Pull Front (11-2) 121

09. Side Bend (13-2) 123

10. Push Up (14-2) 126

11. Scissors In Air (1-3) 129

12. Swan Dive (3-3) 132

13. Leg Pull (4-3) 135

14. Control Balance (5-3) 138

15. Side Kick Kneeling (7-3) 140

Lower Body

01. One Leg Circles (6-1) 143

02. Heel Squeeze Prone (13-1) 145

03. One Side Leg Kick (16-1) 147

04. Side Leg Series (17-1) 150

05. Single Leg Extension (20-1) 153

06. Prone Gluteo (27-1) 155

07. The Bridge (2-2) 157

08. One Leg Kick (4-2) 160

09. Hinge (15-2) 163

10. Rocking (8-3) 165

Upper Body

01. Breast Stroke (2-1) 167

Relax

01. Shell Stretch (22-1) 169

Stretches/Relax

01. Quadriceps (1-E) 171
02. Gluteus Maximus and Quadratus Lumborum (3-E) 171
03. Hamstrings and Calf Muscles 171
04. Gluteus Medius and Sides (4-E) 171
05. Dorsal (5-E) 172
06. Anterior Chain (7-E) 172
07. Pectoral (6-E) 172
08. Posterior Chain (8-E) 172
09. Lateral Chain (9-E) 173
10. Shoulders and Trapezius 173
11. Neck (11-E) 174

Standing Pilates Exercises

01. Ab prep (1-1) 175
02. Breast Stroke (2-1) 176
03. Half Roll Back (4-1) 177
04. Roll Up (5-1) 178
05. One-Leg Circles (6-1) 179
06. Twist (7-1) 180

07. Rolling Like A Ball (8-1) 181
08. One Leg Stretch (9-1) 182
09. Obliques (15-1) 183
10. Scissors (12-1) 184
11. Prone Heel Squeeze (13-1) 185
12. Saw (14-1) 186
13. Oblique Roll-Up (5-1) 187
14. One Side Leg Kick (16-1) 188
15. Side Leg Series, Var. 3 (17-1) 189
16. Single Leg Extension (20-1) 190
17. Shell Stretch (1-1) 191
18. Push Up (14-2) 192
19. Chair (Without Floor Support) 193
20. Split (Without Reference on the Floor) 194
21. Oblique Split (Without Floor Support) 195
22. Back and Forth (Without Floor Support) 196
23. Relevé (Without Floor Support) 197
24. One Leg Kick (4-2) 198
25. Swimming Arms (10-2) 199
26. Side Bend (13-2) 200
27. Swimming (10-2) 201
28. Triceps Kick (Lower Body) 202

2. Tables of Exercises by Goal 203

01. To Strengthen and Reduce the Abdomen 204
02. To Increase Energy 207
03. For The Work Place 210

04. To Improve Everyday Agility 212
  05. For the Shoulders, Back and Chest 215
  06. For the Glutes, Hips, and Legs 218
  07. To Improve Joint Mobility 221
  08. For Back Care 224
  09. For Bedtime 227
  10. For a Pleasant Morning Routine 230

Masterclass **233**

3. Adaptations of exercises to frequent pathologies 234
  01. Common Adaptations 235
  02. Adapted Exercises 242

4. Postural and Functional Assessment 250
  01. Postural Assessment 251
  02. Functional Assessment 259

Annexes 273
  Annex 1. Exercises by Level 274
  Annex 2. Glossary 277
  Annex 3. Bibliography 279

Acknowledgements

To Ana Escobedo for contacting my publisher.

To Marco Pila, my publisher, for making this book a reality.

To Isabel Arechabala for her wonderful illustrations.

To Eva, Ana Isabel, Fer, and Edgar for their dedication during modelling sessions.

To my friends and family for their unconditional support.

To my students for their daily work, which is the source of my experience.

To Eva López for her assistance and for her patience.

Prolog

Compared to countries like the United States, where Pilates schools thrive and spread at astounding speed, the media elsewhere were slower to pick up on the Pilates method, though they now present it as a revelation in mobility disciplines.

Though the medical profession once held that swimming was the best exercise for all patients suffering from back pain and reduced mobility, physicians now regularly recommend Pilates to those same people. Why? What do these two activities have in common? What makes swimming and Pilates different from other forms of exercise?

Swimming is completely impact-free, and it therefore poses absolutely no danger to the joints. In the absence of information about a patient's physical fitness, it is a surefire recommendation for physical activity without risk.

The Pilates method consists of a serie s of exercises, most of them impact-free, which target correct posture, muscle tone, muscle elasticity and articular flexibility with no risk of injury. The muscle groups involved in these exercises are the same ones we all use on a daily basis in both household tasks and in the workplace. It could be said, therefore, that this kind of training has a strong functional component, as both the exercise conditions and the exercises themselves train us to face the challenges of everyday life successfully and free from pain.

At the end of the day, I believe both swimming and Pilates are ideal forms of exercise and that either is to be recommended depending on the practitioner's goals and physical condition. In fact, I would recommend any exercise as long as it meets the following conditions:

- Moderate intensity.
- Frequent
- Programmed
- Good for the joints and muscles
- Good for the mind
- Executed with proper technique.

The method I present in this book can be organized so as to fulfill all of these conditions, but before programming the exercises you need to know them and the basic principles involved in each. This is key to doing the exercises right.

Movement as process: a personal view

Human beings are designed to move, but not any old how. Motion must be orderly, healthy, functional and beneficial, the more the better. As we move, we trigger a chain of processes that improve quality of life if done right, but that cause strain, discomfort and tension if done wrong.

1. As we move, heart rate and body heat increase.
2. The joints begin to warm up and the synovial fluid acts like a grease, allowing the bone structures to slide across one another, instead of grinding painfully together as they move.

3. Ligaments, tendons, menisci, and cartilages are nourished by this movement and respond positively.
4. Exercise produces intense neuromuscular interactions, which build and stimulate the neural pathways required for motion.
5. The more a movement is repeated, the more it will be perfected as the muscles involved become stronger and better coordinated.
6. An active, strong muscle is a healthy muscle that ensures mobility and keeps the associated joints in good fettle.
7. A joint surrounded by active muscles and strong ligaments, tendons, menisci, and cartilages is a healthy joint.

This book explains all of the main Pilates exercises and provides information about the muscles involved in each. It also flags the most common mistakes made in practice and offers variations to allow practitioners to adapt their routines to their own individual needs. Finally, it addresses goals and offers tips, for example to increase your energy levels when you feel listless, to find the ideal bedtime stretch to sleep without backache, or to program the exercises you need to end fatigue and clumsiness during your working day... and so much more.

Why Pilates?

Having seen over the years how the Pilates method works to improve and maintain the health of my students, I am not resigned to watching those who cannot afford the cost or maybe the time required for regular classes to miss out on the benefits of doing the right exercises at the right time. Every day in my studio, I offer guidance on the best exercises for this or that purpose, and it gives me with great pleasure to hear how they work to enhance practitioners' quality of life.

Now I want you to reap the benefits of this revolutionary fitness system. However, you must first understand that there is nothing to gain just by repeating the exercises over and over again, or by going straight to the most advanced exercise in each category. Rather, you need to complete all the steps involved in each exercise properly, rigorously applying the underlying principles of the Pilates method. Otherwise, what you are doing will be merely a somewhat out-there, and possibly harmful, kind of keep-fit.

The relationship between the explanations offered in this book and the need for practitioners of Pilates to gain a thorough understanding of the method is a source of some unease for me, because I am acutely aware that the interpretation of these pages will depend in no small degree on each reader's training experience, and on the extent of their knowledge both of their own bodies and of the Pilates system. I have tried to be as clear as possible and to ensure that positive results will appear from the first, no matter the physical condition or prior experience of the person doing the exercises. Remember that "it is the path to fitness that matters".

Since I cannot personally show readers the exercises or stand by them to oversee their efforts, I cannot be responsible for the results. However, you can contact me by e-mail at vickytimon1971@ gmail.com.

Last but not least, if you have any health issues, you should consult a physician before doing any Pilates exercises.

This book is meant for everyone, regardless of gender, age, physical fitness or experience. This book is meant for you.

Vicky Timón

How to Use This Book

Illustrated muscle structure

The illustrations show in detail the key positions involved in each exercise. Muscle groups colored in red are generally the ones required for movement, although they may also be stabilizing muscles. They are colored red to emphasize their key role in the exercise. Muscles shown in other colors mainly play stabilizing or ancillary roles, while those drawn but not colored are also involved in movement or stabilization, but do not carry out key roles. All muscles must work together as a team, and successful execution of an exercise depends on all of them to achieve the gains pursued.

Even the most simple exercise requires effort, because the question is not merely to do it but to do it well, in depth, keeping good posture, achieving a constant stretch and bilateral balance of the whole body, applying the principles of the Pilates method from the beginning to the end of the exercise.

How To:

This is a description of the exercise, a technical explanation of its execution that explains the different positions illustrated. Under this heading you will find similar remarks to the tips included in the section "Keys to Doing This Exercise Right. The "How To" instructions will help you increase or decrease intensity and achieve the right posture.

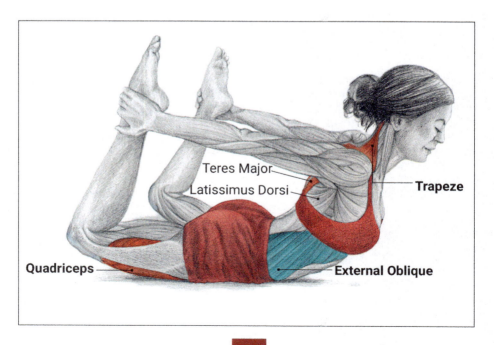

How to Use This Book

Keys to good form

These are verbal or visual tips to help you perform an exercise correctly down to the last detail. They are the keys to success, allowing you to reap the benefits of the exercises. Many of the movements carried out in the Pilates method are potentially harmful and you can hurt yourself by executing the different steps involved incorrectly, due either to bad habits or poor technique. As you practice Pilates, you will learn how to do the exercises right and bad habits affecting movement and posture will gradually disappear from your everyday activity.

Under this same heading, you will also learn how to structure an exercise through breathing. Following the patterns for inhalation and exhalation will help once the exercise is assimilated, especially in the case of complex exercises. In this regard, my advice is to first practice the movement and then learn how to breathe right. In simple exercises it is hardly necessary to think about breathing, since it comes naturally all by itself and one thing does not clash with another. In complex exercises, however, it may take you longer to learn an exercise if you worry too much about proper breathing from the start.

Proper breathing is a cornerstone of the Pilates method and it must be learned,. However, the application of breathing technique to exercises is another matter and it takes time. Once you master it, you will find yourself able to do the exercises with extraordinary fluidity.

Muscles Involved

This section provides an anatomical analysis of the musculature at work while the exercise is carried out. Some muscles produce motion, others stabilize, and a third group assists in supporting or secondary roles. Yet all are important, all must play their role, and all must be properly controlled.

It is exceedingly complicated to show the entire musculature involved in any given exercise. Faced with the need to decide which muscles to show in the anatomical illustrations, I have finally settled on color-coding the most important, which is to say the muscles that really do the work and should therefore feel the strain as you execute the exercise. The others (i.e. muscles not appearing as "key" to an exercise) are detailed under "Others" in "Muscles Involved", generally referring to those that are stretched. Pilates is not a stretching method per se, but stretching is intrinsic to the exercises and, even though it is not the focus of attention it is one of the keys to the spectacular results to be gained from the practice of Pilates.

Benefits and Transferences of Exercise

Knowing why and to what end you are doing an exercise is key information to devising a training program with a clearly-defined goal in mind. This is also a motivation factor because you will eventually look back and realize that exercises that do not obviously show the work you have done have helped you improve your breathing, climb up stairs two by two, lift and carry heavy weights without hurting your back, even perform better at sports.

How to Use This Book

Common mistakes

This section is born of experience; most students fall into these pitfalls sooner or later regardless of their level. Sometimes due to poor technique or out of fatigue, and others just because they are having a bad day... You can minimize such mistakes by keeping your guard up and staying alert.

Adaptations

This book contains a chapter on the use of home Pilates gear and posture modifications in the exercises. Here you will find information to help you resolve issues with pain or discomfort that hamper correct execution. These adaptations are for the most part surprisingly simple.

Variations

Under this heading, you will find exercises similar to the main one but with more or less intensity, and/or including another muscle group. These are as interesting as the principal exercises of the method and you should make sure to master them too. Variations are an excellent way to avoid routine and boredom.

Annotations

These are nuggets of information that are included to clarify some exercises, including specific instructions for execution and general remarks about the patterns of movement involved in exercises.

Classification of exercises

This book proposes a classification of exercises into upper body, lower body, mixed, abdominals, and relaxation/stretches, which differs from the conventional ranking by level. However, the level of each exercise and other key information are included in the heading.

"Abdominal," "Lower Body," "Upper Body," "Mixed," and "Stretches/Relax" are the five categories you will find. The work classified as "Abdominal" mainly relates to the four abdominal muscle groups, although other muscles may also be involved. However, the abdominal muscles also play an important role in all of the other categories except "Stretches/Relax".

- Example: "ABDOMINAL. Slow Double Leg Stretch (1-2)." "ABDOMINAL:" Category to which the exercise belongs, although the name rather suggests a lower-body exercise.
- "Slow Double Leg Stretch:" Name of the exercise. These names should be taken with a grain of salt, since not all schools of Pilates employ the same nomenclature. The translation of this work employs the English

How to Use This Book

names of the exercises that the author learned at the Stott and Polestar schools.

- "1-2:" The classification of each exercise by difficulty involves three levels. This numbering would therefore refer to exercise 1 of the second, or medium, level. It is important to know what kind of exercise you are doing, because you may sometimes encounter unexpected difficulties. Such problems may many different roots, including poor muscle tone, the need to maintain the base principles of the method, lack of strength, balance or endurance, deficient spinal flexibility, aerial exercises, and so forth. For instance, "Swimming" is a relatively easy level 2 exercise, yet no one would say so at first sight. The complexity in "swimming" lies in the need to stretch the spine and the demand for abdominal support while performing a movement that almost everyone tends to shorten. If you do not (or cannot) stretch your spine enough, your lower back zone will be overloaded: avoiding this pitfall requires experience and practice commensurate with level 2.

As you read through the exercises you can also scan the QR codes with your phone or open the short URL links in your computer in order to watch the videos and better understand how to perform them.

Illustration

Keys to good form

Main Exercise

How To

Adaptations

Variations

Notes

Tips and common mistakes

Illustration of Variations

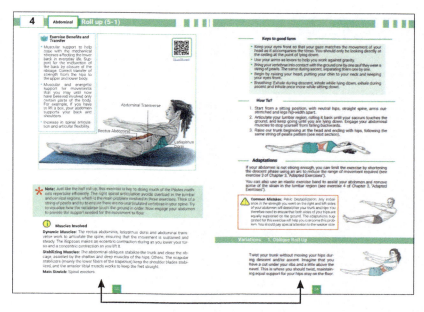

This book is meant to be read as a double-spread manual.

At the foot of the page, one can find a series of exercises continuing on to the facing page.

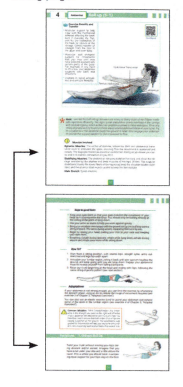

In eBook format, the book is presented vertically, so that the main exercise can be found on the first, even-numbered page; and its different variations on the second, odd-numbered page.

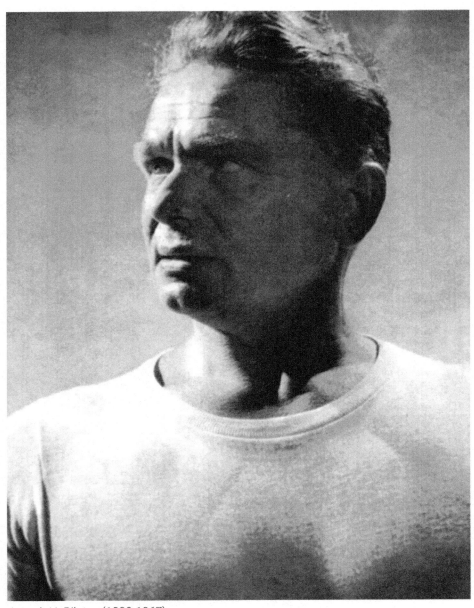
Joseph H. Pilates (1880-1967)

Introducing the Pilates Method

Historical background

Joseph H. Pilates said: "In 10 sessions you'll feel the difference, in 20 sessions you'll see the difference, and in 30 sessions you'll have a whole new body."

Pilates himself did not enjoy particularly good health as a child and he was far from athletic. He was the loser in schoolboy fights and he would come in last in races. When his classmates had recovered from their exertions he still hurt all over. He was scrawny, even sickly, and he suffered from rickets. However, his physical limitations drove him to try all kinds of sports, learning the best of each and designing numerous exercises that are still used in therapeutic gymnastics to this day: he was a true researcher of mobility.

The outbreak of World War I found him working in England and he interned in a concentration camp. The war provided Pilates with a testbed in which to develop and hone his knowledge of mobility and muscular balance, working as a medic with injured German prisoners. Even those unable to stand benefitted from the method devised by Pilates, who installed springs on their beds so that they could work with resistance to strengthen their muscles. As these patients grew stronger their mobility improved, which in turn ensured a better and faster recovery.

After the war, the German army offered him a permanent position as a physical instructor in 1926, but he declined, preferring to go to the USA, where he founded his first studio, whose clients included a clutch of celebrity dancers, including George Balanchine, Ruth Saint Denis, Ted Shawn and Martha Graham. His own fame skyrocketed; everyone wanted to train with Pilates or learn from him. The Pilates Method (then called "Contrology") quickly became a model for conscious mobility techniques designed to develop muscular and postural control, and to enhance flexibility, elasticity, agility, endurance/muscle resistance and power. His studio was filled with patients from Lenox Hill Hospital, sent by its Orthopedics ward.

The Pilates Method was beginning to take shape as a successful commercial product, though it remained as yet beyond the reach of any but the well-heeled.

The original exercises that Pilates described in his notes require excellent technique, reflecting the demands he placed on his pupils. Nowadays, Pilates manuals generally offer a compendium of exercises classified according to their levels of difficulty and performance. Each Pilates school is different and adds its own personal touch, though always respecting the main principles of execution. These principles are the nexus for all the tangled webs of emerging trends in conscious mobility tat now crowd the market.

Today, film, music and sports stars like Madonna, Julia Roberts, Brad Pitt, Michael Jordan and Uma Thurman to name but a few regularly practice Pilates and are always quick to extol the virtues of the method, because they more than anyone earn their living from their physique. These celebrities consistently describe Pilates is a key therapy for health, strength, and beauty.

The good news is that the Pilates method is nowadays no longer the preserve of actors and dancers but has come within everybody's reach in fitness centers and facilities everywhere.

The bad news is that the method has now been so widely marketed that anyone can feel like an instructor after a six-hour training seminar that barely provides time to grasp the basic principles.

A Radical Change

When I learned the basic principles of the Pilates method something changed in my understanding of movement and, by extension, in my approach to teaching fitness. Whoever feels the way I felt, whether teacher or student, will never be the same again. This might seem like an exaggeration, but it is the only way I can explain what happened to me.

I thought I was in peak physical condition and that I would have no difficulty learning Pilates given my experience in the fitness world. That was not how it turned out however. I had to make a huge effort to break with ingrained faulty patterns of movement. I had no idea how to use the deep fibers in my abdomen (transverse abdominal muscle), or how to breathe right, and I trembled like a leaf whenever I had to repeat the same abdominal exercise eight times while trying not to move my hips. The explanation for this is not that I was unfit, but rather that I was only fit "on the outside." My dynamic muscles were very strong, but my static or postural muscles were weak because I had never used them consciously, never thought of the importance of maintaining the right posture during training. I was only interested in lifting more weight or increasing my reps, but (and here's the key!) I had never been aware of the importance of maintaining good posture throughout every step and action of the day.

The Pilates method has now become a part of my mobility and it will stay with me for the rest of my life. Bad posture in whatever shape or form now makes me uncomfortable. My postural muscles now automatically work this way, and by training I constantly discipline and remind, so that they now work almost without conscious effort on my part. Long story short, I am able to save and I find myself feeling better than ever before, entirely free of discomfort or pain. Who could ask for more?

This is why I believe that techniques of this kind will always be relevant. The Pilates method offers an excellent base for mobility and, even though new techniques and training systems may be created, good posture will always be key to keeping our joints healthy. Pilates invented and shaped one of the safest, most efficient and beneficial exercise methods in the history of fitness.

General Benefits of Fitness

Well-programmed workouts with the right levels of control, frequency and intensity produce numerous benefits in the body. Each individual is unique and therefore exercise affects different people in different ways, but it always brings health, energy and a positive outlook because programmed training increases the activity of hormones like adrenalin, serotonin and oxytocin, which improve mood, produce feelings of well-being and can even increase sex drive.

As mentioned, exercise produces the following benefits, among others:

- Increased self-esteem, self-confidence and mental performance
- Improved psychological states and prevention of anxiety and depression
- Reduced stress and tension
- Increased energy and vitality
- Improved general physical condition
- Increased longevity and quality of life
- Reduced risk of high blood pressure, diabetes, obesity, osteoporosis, bone decalcification, insomnia, colon cancer, etc.
- Increased metabolic rate
- Improved cholesterol levels
- Increased secretion of growth hormone
- Increased blood flow to the brain, which in turn increases alertness
- Better digestion
- Stronger immune system

Particular Benefits of Pilates

Physical	Mental
Increased flexibility	Improved mental health
Increased elasticity	Higher self-esteem
Greatly improved agility	Lower stress levels
Increased functional strength	Better sleep
Increased physical health	Improved sex life
Recovery of mobility	Aumento de la confianza
Improved mobility	Better concentration
Lower risk of injury	Longer attention span
Enhanced physical awareness (proprioception)	
Improved balance	
Breathing control	
Better posture	
Reduced joint pain, muscle fatigue and inflammation	

Exercises by Category

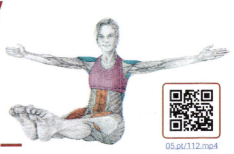

05.pt/112.mp4

— **Introduction to the Exercises** —

In this book you will find a compendium of exercises, classified according to the region of the body worked. The Pilates method rests basically on preparation of the abdomen spread energy, support the back and generally stabilize movements throughout the body.

Even though the abdomen is always the primary focus of attention, energy must also be spread to other regions of the . Therefore the exercises are classified as "Abdominal," "Mixed," "Upper Body," "Lower Body," "Relax" plus an extra chapter on "Stretches".

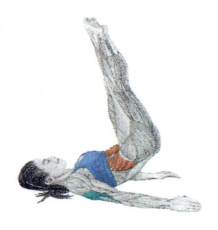

Aside from this classification by bodily region, you will also learn the level of each exercise, which will allow you to devise a training plan based on progression of difficulty.

Both of these classifications (by region and by difficulty) are included in the table of contents at the beginning of this book.

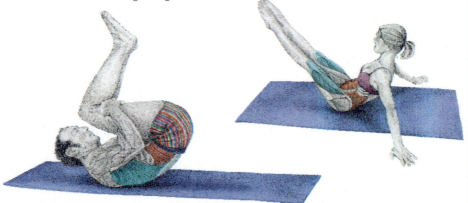

Basic Principles

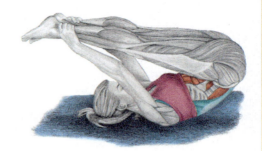

Introduction

Learning the principles of the method and applying them systematically is key to reaping the rewards. If you can automate these techniques, you will have learned how to stay healthier for the rest of your lifetime. It is no exaggeration to say that life will never be the same when you master these principles, because your mobility and perception of posture will have changed.

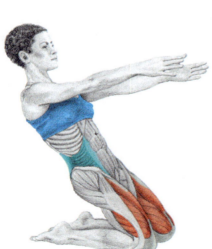

These principles vary in name and number in different Pilates schools, but in practice, they are in fact always fundamentally the same, because there is no other way to assimilate the method, which loses its virtue if it is not properly taught.

In order to understand the potential of these exercises, you must first learn their underlying principles. These are the basis of the method, and without them, any apparatus will be merely a platform with springs and hooks of the kind that you might find in the weights room of a well-equipped gym or in any ordinary keep-fit class.

Introduction

Visual Images

It is easier to learn the Pilates method using visual guides in the form of mental images suggested by the instructor to help students achieve clear, efficient movements. Most people already hold some images of this kind in their heads, although they are sometimes misconceived, causing tensions and bad postural habits and potentially leading to injury and other physical deviations. The key to success in Pilates lies in modifying existing images and incorporating new ones. For instance, someone seeking to separate their shoulders from their ears by stretching their neck forwards would only increase their kyphosis or "hunchback" posture, overloading the upper back and risking spasms and soreness in the neck muscles and trapezius.

The different parts of the body are activated by neural pathways, hence the importance of visualizations. For instance, it is easier to raise your arm by imagining an outstretched index finger than an outstretched pinkie finger.

You will find the visualization guidelines you need in the sections headed "Keys to Assimilating the Principle of...," included in the following discussion of the basic Pilates principles, and under "Keys to Good Form," presented with every exercise in this book. If you try the exercises while visualizing the guideline images, you will find them much easier to perform.

Principles Discussed in this Book

1. Cranio-vertebral articulation
2. Scapular stabilization
3. Pelvic stabilization
4. Axial elongation
5. Bodily alignment and balance
6. Breathing
7. Integration

The Abdominal Connection

Connecting your rectus abdominis, your transverse abdominal muscle and your abdominal oblique muscles will improve the health of your back, since these muscles are key to stabilizing the hips and elongating the spine, and they control the opening and closing of the thorax.

Principles of the Pilates Method

Whenever a reference to abdominal musculature occurs in this book, the term connection will be used more often than muscular contraction, since the goal is to keep the muscles of the abdomen working throughout a lengthy stretch of time. Connection allows you to do this without overloading. To better understand this, picture a typical biceps curl, an exercise that involves gripping a weight in the hand, flexing the elbow is flexed and lifting. More or less strength is exerted depending on the weight used and this will in turn affect the intensity with which the biceps contracts, since their can be no lift without contraction. In the case of the abdomen two kinds of kinds of effort may be required: on one hand, exercises that use sporadic contractions to flex the torso, just like in the preceding example and as in, conventional abdominal exercises; and, on the other, exercises that demand abdominal connection to hold a given posture. This kind of effort is present in all Pilates exercises, even those that also include contractions.

Superficial View

Deep View

Quadratus Lumborum

External Oblique Minor

Rectus Abdominis

External Oblique Major

Transverse Abdominal

Rectus Abdominis (cross-section)

1 Cranio-Vertebral Articulation

The head must move according to the action performed, and the gaze must accompany the movement. If either of these two factors does not match the action, the muscles of the neck and upper back will be overloaded, which can lead to serious injury, such as slipped disks. For this reason, the movements made must be gestures that are carried out need to be well-coordinated and harmonious. The head-neck structure is of the utmost importance to attain this goal.

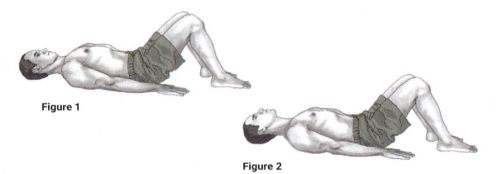

Figure 1

Figure 2

Benefits of Cranio-Vertebral Articulation

- It increases the flow and distribution of energy, diminishing and even eliminating headaches, tension and cervical overload.
- It eliminates negative motion patterns and injurious postures of the head-neck structure.
- It ensures a good distribution of energy between the head, shoulders and spine.

Keys to Assimilating the Principle of Cranio-Vertebral Articulation

- Visual Image: put your chin close to your Adam's apple and lengthen the back of your neck, trying to touch the wall with the middle part of your skull.
- When you are lying on your back and want to get up, put your chin close to your throat and bring your gaze to the front from the start.
- Flatten your chin and relax your throat.
- Imagine that somebody is pulling your head back from behind, stretching your neck.
- Breathe out emptying your chest of air. Now relax your chest and align your head on the same axis as your spine is (normally a little further back).

Principles of the Pilates Method

Exercises to Practice This Principle

- Lie on your back with your arms by your sides, keeping your shoulders away from your ears. Now raise and lower your chin moving only the last vertebra in contact with your skull. The rest of your vertebrae should remain motionless (Figures 1 and 2).

- Sit cross-legged and then stretch your spine upwards as if you wanted to touch the ceiling with the crown of your skull. Without losing this stretch, flex your head forwards and back, then sideways to left and right, and then in circles, bringing together all of the previous movements (see Figure 3-6).

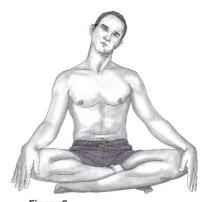

Figure 3

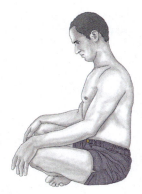

Figure 4

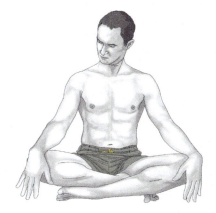

Figure 5

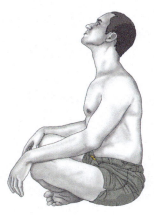

Figure 6

2 Scapular Stabilization

Exertion of the face, neck and shoulders increase tension in the shoulder girdle, neck and the back of your head. Scapular stabilization work will help you focus on your head, shoulders, shoulder blades, collarbone and chest.

This principle seeks to ensure correct positioning of the shoulders, which should stay neither too high nor too lower, away from the ears, and set back in a relaxed posture. The shoulder blades should glide up and down, inward and outward in broad sweeps. Among the countless possible positions, the right one will always be the most neutral, pointing downward and inward.

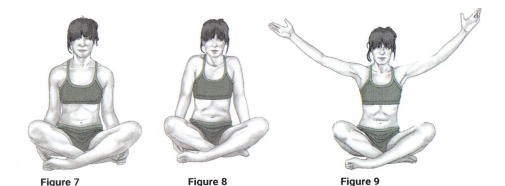

Figure 7   Figure 8   Figure 9

Benefits of Scapular Stabilization

- Improved neural stimulation of the muscles in the shoulders and thoracic region (rotator cuff, thoracic vertebrae, costovertebral joints and intercostal muscles).
- Improved oxygen exchange and easier breathing.
- Improved proprioception of shoulder and chest muscles.
- Improved transfer of strength towards head, arms and spine.
- Reduced risk of cervical injuries and overload, headaches and shoulder injuries.

Keys to Assimilating the Principle of Scapular Stabilization

Visual Image: Shoulders away from the ears and pointing back.

- Lower your shoulder blades towards the back pockets of your pants.
- Breathe out to empty your chest of air.
- Feel your back muscles activate.
- Try to bring your shoulder blades together in the small of your back, then relax the muscles concerned.

Principles of the Pilates Method

Exercises to Practice this Principle

- Seated cross-legged, raise and lower your shoulders until you find a neutral position with your shoulders away from your ears (Figures 7 and 8).
- Seated cross-legged, make circles with your arms while keeping your shoulders away from your ears (Figure 9).
- Lying on your back with your knees up, raise your shoulders towards the ceiling and then try to touch the floor with them. Keep your shoulders away from your ears throughout (Figure 10).
- Lying on your back, move your shoulder blades forward and back, towards and away from the wall (Figure 11).
- Lying on your back with arms outstretched in a cross, bring your hands together over your chest and then separate them, bringing your arms back down to the floor (Figure 12).
- Stand or sit with your arms outstretched like a cross keeping your shoulders away from your ears. Stretch your arms outwards as if you were trying to touch the walls on each side while stretching your head upwards toward the ceiling (Figure 13).

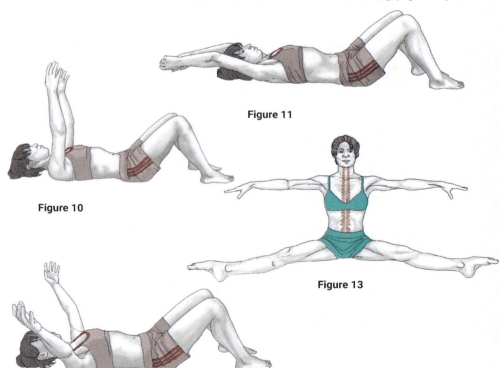

Figure 11

Figure 10

Figure 13

Figure 12

3   Pelvic Stabilization

The concept of pelvic stabilization is based on the neutral position of the hips. The goal is to ensure that the triangle formed by the ASIS (Anterior superior iliac spine) and the pubic symphysis stays parallel to the floor when you are in a lying or supine position and is aligned between the ceiling and the floor when the person is sitting or standing. Neutral hips prevent articular stress in the lower back (lumbar region).

When the hips are placed in the neutral position, it is normal for a hollow to appear between the lumbar region and the floor when you are lying on your back. This feeling can be a little scary if you are injured or suffer from chronic lower back pain, but this is actually nothing to the old, mistaken belief that this structural lumbar curve is somehow a problem. Everybody has a structural curve of this kind and you need to learn to respect it when you do Pilates exercises. Any discomfort you may feel in this area will gradually fade away over time.

Benefits of Pelvic Stabilization

- It relieves stress in the lower back region during exercises in which the trunk/torso is flexed and extended.
- It ensures correct absorption of bodyweight on the lumbar curve.
- It helps with dissociation in exercises for articulation of the legs and spine.
- It allows steady toning of the deep lower muscles of the abdomen (abdominal transverse).
- It ensures correct distribution of energy between the abdominal oblique muscles, the rectus abdominis and the abdominal transverse muscles.

Keys to Assimilate the Principle of Pelvic Stabilization

Visual Image: Your hips should feel centered and not pushed back or forwards when you stand. Lying down, your hips should feel relaxed resting on the floor, allowing a gentle lumbar curve to appear.

1. Empty your chest of air to eliminate tension in the middle and upper back, so that you can position your hips better.
2. Unblock your knees.
3. Respect the lumbar curve.

Principles of the Pilates Method

Importance of Stabilization

Stabilizations give sense to the Pilates method. Stabilization underpins the Pilates method, marking the difference between a well-executed exercise and a mediocre one. It is this detail that makes the exercises beneficial for health and fitness than rather a potential cause of cause of injury or a mere pastime which will eventually be dropped out of boredom.

Failure to stabilize your hips during any exercise, for example dancing for hours at a party, causes lower back pain. This is because the lower back muscles are subject to a lot of strain. However, if the abdominal muscles are voluntarily activated in these circumstances, the workload is shared and any pain that you do feel will quickly fade.

The same happens with your shoulders: there are many situations that can cause bad posture, including cold, shyness, anger, working at a computer and carrying heavy weights, and the usual reaction is to raise your shoulders and roll them forwards, putting additional strain on the trapezius, which leads to overload and muscular spasms and discomfort. Keeping your shoulders away from your ears and adopting an "elegant" pose prevents this overload.

Training, repetition, thinking through the exercises as you do them, modifying the postures that cause overload, awareness of bad postural habits and making the effort to change and to adopt the new habits learned are the keys to a healthy and attractive body.

Most Pilates exercises are done lying on the floor, in a continuous struggle against gravity. From this position, arms, trunk and legs are moved, always upwards. This extra effort must be supported by the abdominals, which form a major muscle group, lest the back should suffer.

Testing yourself and successfully overcoming problems requires training. This is one of the reasons why the Pilates method is divided into levels of difficulty, not to be confused with levels of intensity. The latter can be attained by means of any exercise present in this book from the very beginning, but difficulty can only be overcome through continuous training and progression through different levels of expertise. A difficult exercise can only be successfully performed after an easier one is mastered.

By "success" we mean the attainment of health benefits, increased physical fitness and enhanced proprioception. In the specific case of pelvic stabilization, success takes the form of greater abdominal strength to support of the lower back.

3 Pelvic Stabilization

Exercises to Practice this Principle

Move your hips forwards, backwards and into the neutral position from a seated position. Neutral is the correct position, but pushing at both extremes will help you become more aware of the positions to avoid as a matter of a postural habit (Figures 14 and 15).

"Cat" and "horse" poses: On all fours, arch and extend your spine and then flex it downwards, paying more attention to the position of your hips than to the articulation of your upper back (Figures 16 and 17).

In a standing position, push your hips forwards and then pull them backwards, seeking to restore the neutral position of your hips after each repetition(Figures 18 and 19).

In a standing position, flex your hips to left and right, seeking to restore the neutral position of your hips after each repetition (Figures 20 and 21).

Lying on your back, flex one of your knees and then let it drop sideways to the floor. Finish by sliding the leg back in line with the other until it is completely straight.(Figures 22-24).

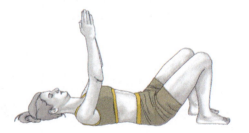

Figure 14

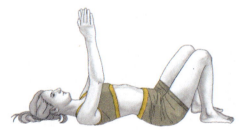

Figure 15

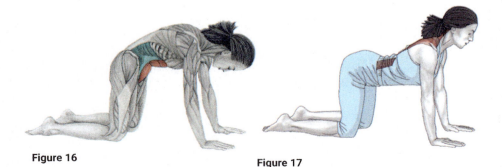

Figure 16

Figure 17

Principles of the Pilates Method

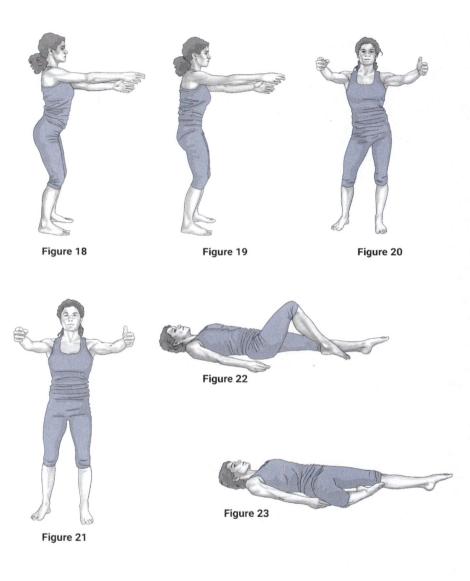

Figure 18

Figure 19

Figure 20

Figure 21

Figure 22

Figure 23

Figure 24

4   Axial Elongation

Elongating the spine consists of feeling your back stretch and grow from the base of your skull down to your sacral region as the vertebrae separate from each other, softening and nourishing the intervertebral discs.

Meanwhile, articulating the spine means moving each of vertebrae needed in order safely and efficiently to perform the exercises one by one. Articulating the spine without axial elongation can cause vertebral shear, however, resulting in injury to the vertebrae themselves and to the intervertebral discs, circulatory system and nervous system. Both Pilates exercises and by extension everyday activity demand a range of different movements involving the spine. In this light, it is very important to be aware of the localization and direction of the movements concerned.

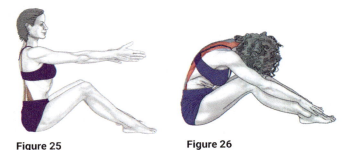

Figure 25   Figure 26

Benefits of Axial Elongation

- It helps segment movement and avoids compressive and shearing forces on the spine.
- It improves proprioception by dissociation of movements made by the limbs.
- It increases spinal mobility.
- It allows functional re-education in all positions, helping you learn how to move and position yourself, so that repeated and routine gestures do not cause injury.

Keys to Assimilating the Axial Elongation Principle

Visual Image: imagine your vertebrae separating one from the next as your stretch your spine up towards the ceiling .

1. Stretch your spine upwards until you can feel "air" between your vertebrae.
2. Seek an elegant pose, without "hunching" your back (kyphosis), keeping your shoulders away from your ears and maintaining abdominal connection.
3. Lying on your back, let your hips rest against the floor, allowing a hollow to appear between your lower back and the floor, and stretch your torso.

Principles of the Pilates Method

Exercises to Practice this Principle

Seated on the floor with your legs apart to the width of your hips and your knees gently flexed, flex your trunk forwards while gliding your hands down your shins to your feet, breathing out as you do so. Breathe in and return to the sitting position stretching out your spine vertebra by vertebra, as if you were trying to touch the ceiling with the crown of your head (Figures 25 and 26).

Stand with your knees slightly bent and your arms spread out in a cross and flex your trunk from side to side without moving your hips or legs (Figure 27).

Standing with gently flexed knees to avoid blocking, flex and stretch out your spine vertebra by vertebra as if you were trying to touch the ceiling with the crown of your head (Figures 28 and 29).

Lying on your back, try to touch the wall behind you with the crown of your head (Figure 30).

Do Level 1 abdominal exercise "Ab Prep" (Figures 31 and 32).

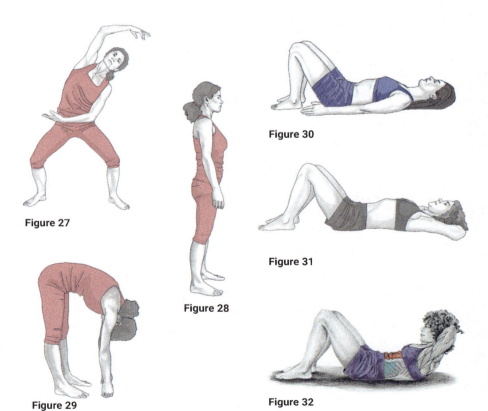

Figure 27

Figure 28

Figure 29

Figure 30

Figure 31

Figure 32

5 Abdominal Connection

Connecting the rectus abdominis, transverse and oblique muscles improves back health, because these muscles play a key role in stabilizing the hips, elongating the spine and controlling the opening and closure of the chest.

When referring to abdominal muscles, I use the word "connection" much more often than "contraction," because the goal is to keep the muscles in your abdomen working over a considerable lapse of time, as if they were postural muscles. Connection allows this while avoiding overload.

We may distinguish two different kinds of abdominal work consisting of steady contractions to flex the trunk, as in conventional abs exercises (sit-ups, ab prep), and the abdominal connection required to maintain a posture. Effort of the latter kind is present in every exercise, including those that also include contractions.

When you connect your abdomen, it flattens and hardens, and you can see and feel how your waistline is reduced.

Benefits of Abdominal Connection

- Improved protection of the lumbar region.
- Support for the abdominal organs.
- Improved spinal elongation.
- Improved head-to-tail transfer of energy.
- Stronger abdominal muscles from the inside out.

Keys to Assimilating the Abdominal Connection Principle

Visual Image: Close your ribcage as if about to cough, relax your back while keeping the muscular action you have attained, stop any urge to urinate or defecate and tuck your navel inward.

1. Lying down, imagine that you have to harden and flatten your abdomen because the ceiling is about to fall down on you.
2. Standing in front of a mirror, open your ribs as if you were trying to tuck your belly in and out, then shut your ribcage, flattening your abdomen. The second pose is the right one.
3. Imagine that someone is about to punch you in the belly and you have to protect yourself keeping it hard, without arching your back.

Principles of the Pilates Method

Exercises to practice this principle

Basic Abdominal Exercise or Ab Prep. You will learn how to clase your ribcage as you raise your trunk and how to keep your ribcage shut as you lower it. The ribcage should never open during exercises, although you of course have to open it outside practice.

Superman. Take careto keep your belly tucked in and lock your lower ribs while doing this exercise.

Whenever you are doing Pilates exercises or making any other short exertion that does not require significant ventilation, like pushing a couch, carrying a heavy load for a while or doing anything that requires a one-off effort.

In situations like walking, office working, aerobic sports and so on you should try to leave your ribcage open but your navel connected. This dissociation is complex, but you will succeed by practice and training. Don't give up or get frustrated if you don't succeed at first, because this trick takes a while to master. You need to shut your sphincters as if you were gently holding back the need to urinate or defecate as you tuck your navel inward, but at the same time you must let your ribcage open and close normally as your breathe.

This is because we need to breathe deeply in order to keep fit. The diaphragm is a muscle that splits us in two right under the ribs. As we breathe in, the diaphragm drops and pushes down on the digestive, urinary and reproductive organs; as we breathe out, it rises, pressing up on the heart and the lungs. These "pressures" are a necessary part of your physiology, and if you try to cancel them out you will fall sick.

Complete and deep breathing is key, do not try to prevent. In fact, the more often you breathe like this the better.

6 Body Alignment and Balance

Aligning your arms, legs and head requires a subtle internal effort, because we all gradually acquire bad habits that put this alignment out of whack. These might include tilting your head to the side, treading with the outer part of the foot or walking with your feet turned outwards.

Achieving muscular balance on both sides of the body also requires a conscious effort, because we grow used to doing some tasks with our right hand and others with our left, to always using the same leg to step over obstacles using the same leg, and so on.

Working with the Pilates method, you can try to realign your body segments and equalize strength on both sides. Success will improve your structural and muscular balance. Pilates does not admit one-sided work but seeks the same intensity on both sides of the body work, but this can only happen if you set this goal consciously. As time goes by, these gestures will become automatic and will hardly need any effort.

Poor balance due to corporal misalignment interrupts energy flows and hampers the correct use of strength by the body as a whole and in the segments involved in a given exercise.

Benefits of Abdominal Connection

- Correct energy transfer in strength chains
- Less chance of injuries due to overload on any one side
- Improved posture postural patterns
- Economy of effort during motion
- Reduction in injuries and strains
- ds

Keys to Assimilating the Abdominal Connection Principle

1. Keep both hips and both shoulders at the same height.
2. Think about your weaker, non-dominant side: it should work as hard as the stronger side.
3. Visualize both sides of your body as you do each exercise.
4. Spread your energy all around your body without leaving any part relaxed or slack.
5. One-sidedness is a bad habit. Avoid it!

Principles of the Pilates Method

Exercises to Practice this Principle

- Squats to work on lower body balance. From a standing position, bend your knees as if you were going to sit down on a low stool, flexing at the hip so that your knees come no further forward than your toes as you squat (Figures 33 and 34).
- Half roll with elastic exercise band to work on full body balance. Sitting with your legs out straight about hip-width apart and slightly flexed knees, articulate your hips and lower back/lumbar region, rounding them, then reverse the process to return to the neutral position (Figure 35).
- Biceps in half roll with exercise band to work on upper body balance. Do a half roll and hold the position while you flex and extend your elbows, working against the resistance of the band (Figure 36).

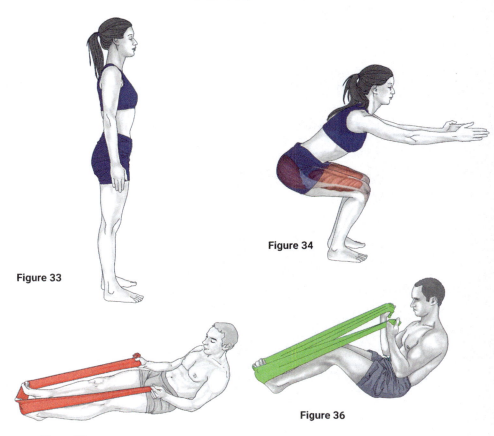

Figure 33

Figure 34

Figure 35

Figure 36

7 Breathing

Breathing is as important to the proper execution of Pilates exercises as any of the other principles discussed in this chapter, although it gets a lot more press as the best-known facet of the method.

Breathing correctly as you do your exercises is important because it helps with execution and good form. However, in trying to maintain proper breathing, we may sometimes forget other principles that are equally important. If you cannot follow a given breathing pattern and do an exercise with good form, the best thing to do is to breathe as best you can until you have completely mastered the mechanics of exercise and only then apply the required breathing pattern. When you do, you will feel how everything flows more smoothly with good form.

Pilates Breathing Is completely conscious

It is impossible to breathe this way unconsciously, because the muscles involved in Pilates breathing are dynamic, and they would become exhausted if they had to work all day.

This conscious breathing tones the intercostal muscles, the serrates, the movement of the diaphragm in parallel to the ground (opening and closing the ribcage) and the abdominal muscles.

Benefits of Breathing

- It orders movement.
- It helps with scapular stabilization.
- It improves spinal articulation.
- Exhalation helps with abdominal connection.
- It enhances your concentration as you do the exercises.

Keys to Assimilating the Breathing Principle

1. Breathe out gently so that you would only cause a candle flame to flicker as you empty your chest of air.
2. Keep your abdomen and your chest still as you breathe.
3. Breathe in gently without raising your shoulders to your ears.
4. Breathe in the air needed for the activity you are doing, neither more nor less.
5. As a general rule, breathe out during the stage of an exercise that demands the most effort.

Principles of the Pilates Method

How To Breathe

Expand your the ribs outwards to the sides as you inhale and close them as you breathe out. The best way to feel this movement is by placing your hands on either side of your ribcage. Your abdomen and your chest should not move as you breathe, so you will not need too much air.

This way of breathing helps with scapular stabilization, closure of the ribcage, abdominal connection and neutral hip positioning.

Thoracic breathing raises the chest and overloads the upper back, while abdominal breathing results in lax posture as the abdominal muscles are necessarily slackened. However, this does not mean that we should stop breathing thoracically or abdominally; on the contrary, both are necessary but at different times depending on your activity.

The Right Breathing for each Activity

You cannot breathe as described if you are running, because in these conditions the body demands much more oxygen than you can provide only by expanding the ribcage sideways, and you will have to expand it upwards as well.

Likewise, you cannot breathe like this while sleeping, because the abdomen is the part of the body that moves the most during sleep. Other sports also require their own breathing patterns.

Pilates breathing is therefore only to be used when you are doing Pilates exercises.

Notice that the diaphragm, the flat muscle that splits us in two under the ribs, is designed to move not only sideways but also up and down. However, this movement is not used in Pilates breathing. If you consciously override any of the diaphragm's natural movements, it will stop squeezing and moving your internal organs, with potentially dire results on the proper functioning of organs like the stomach.

7 Breathing

Exercises to Practice this Principle

- Place your hands on either side of your ribcage to feel it expand sideways as you breathe in. As you exhale, imagine that you are trying to make your ribs touch at the pit of your stomach (Figure 37).
- Lie on your back and breathe so that it is not obvious that you are doing so but without starving yourself of air (Figure 38).
- Sit with your legs hip-width apart and your knees half flexed. Now lower your trunk forwards, relax your arms along your legs and breathe, carrying the air upwards towards back (Figure 39).
- Do the Level 1 abdominal exercise "Hundred" (Figure 40).
- Breathe with your chest, keeping your abdomen still (Figure 41).
- Breathe with your abdomen, keeping your chest still (Figure 42).
- Stand with your legs wider than shoulder-width apart and raise and lower your arms, crossing them in front of you and behind you (Figures 43 and 44).)

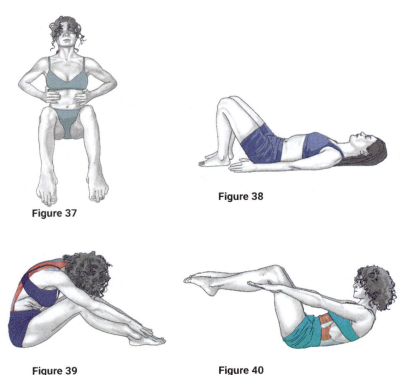

Figure 37

Figure 38

Figure 39

Figure 40

Principles of the Pilates Method

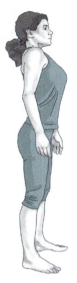

Figure 41

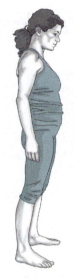

Figure 42

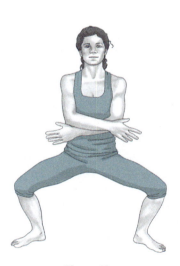

Figure 43

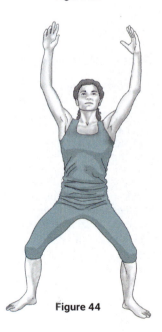

Figure 44

8 Integration and Control

Integration means doing Pilates exercises efficiently and with fluidity and economy of effort. Once this goal is attained, what you have learned will be transferred to your everyday activities and you will become less prone to injury caused repetitive movements and sudden reactions.

Orderly movement will not transmit feelings of strain but rather of efficiency. Tension decreases in the area stabilized and we "feel" the movement as freer and lighter, almost ethereal.

All physical learning is attained by training, repeating an action so that it becomes entirely familiar and can be easily reproduced. This process will be more or less difficult and take more or less time depending on the athletic habits that you have acquired over the course of your life.

The automatization of movements leaves an imprint and this imprint can be made permanent, but efficiency and economy of effort are lost as a result of long periods of inactivity.

Tip: A difficult exercise done any old how will not provide any benefits and it could lead to injury. Never forget that the path leading to the exercise is more important than the exercise itself.

What is integration?

Our goal is to succeed in transferring the patterns of movement learned by doing Pilates exercises to our everyday actions. Pilates is a process of continuous learning, and you must understand that the exercises are done not only to work out and keep fit, which would be contrary to the underlying the philosophy of the method. Transference is a key aspect of the Pilates method, and a section with the title "Exercise Benefits and Transfer" will be found on most pages.

Lifting a large plant pot, climbing stairs, sitting eight hours at a desk, doing household chores or holding a baby are all actions that demand effort from both superficial and deep muscles, resilience and, above all, good posture. Pilates exercises do not reproduce these actions as such, but they do work on the elements that will allow you to perform them with strength, comfort and safety, three factors that converge in a single word: health.

Principles of the Pilates Method

Kinetic Chains

Closed kinetic chains use both the hands and feet for support. They therefore require less motion control because they allow little freedom of movement. Exercises of this kind therefore fire postural reflexes and it is easier to learn or train new patterns of movement.

In this light, we may begin with closed-chain exercises and, once these are learned, move on to open or semi-open kinetic chain exercises. A clear example would be arching your back and flexing your spine: this drill is very difficult to assimilate from a standing position, but it is easily understood on all fours, with hands and knees planted firmly on the ground.

The four-stage process of acquiring motor skills

1. Subconscious inability: the student knows nothing at all about the exercise or drill taught..
2. Conscious inability: the student is aware that she/he does not know how to perform an exercise.
3. Conscious ability: the student knows that she/he can do the exercise and control the movements required with effort.
4. Subconscious ability: the student has integrated the knowledge and skills taught, which she/he can now assimilate into daily activity.

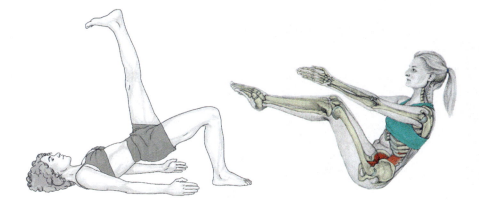

Principles of the Pilates Method

Keys to Assimilating the Integration and Control Principle

- Control of pelvic motion on all planes.
- Recreation of images of motion like "light," "elegant," "open..."
- Analytically, all the keys previously used.

Exercises to Practice this Principle

MIXED Level 2 exercise "Side Bend." Figure 45

LOWER-BODY Level 2 Exercise "Bridge, Variation 1." Figure 46

ABDOMINAL Level 2 Exercise "Teaser, Variation 2." Figure 47

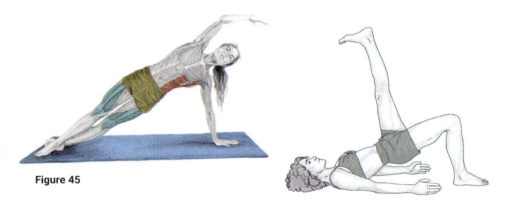

Figure 45

Figure 46

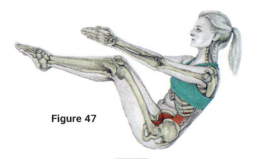

Figure 47

1 Abdominal — Ab Prep (1-1)

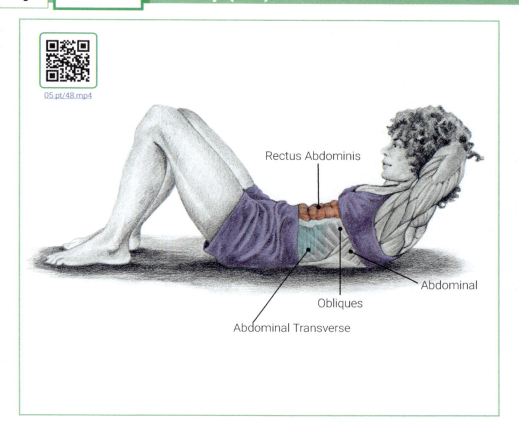

05.pt/48.mp4

- Rectus Abdominis
- Abdominal Obliques
- Abdominal Transverse

Exercise Benefits and Transfer

- Muscular support to help cope with the mechanical stresses affecting the lower back in everyday life.
- Support for the midsection of the back as a result of closing the ribcage.
- Correct transfer of strength from the hips to the upper and lower body.
- Muscular and energetic support for movements that you may until now have believed involved only certain parts of the body. For example, if you have to lift a box, your abdomen supports your back and shoulders.
- Learning the right way to do the most common exercises used in gyms.

Keys to good form

- Look straight ahead. When you are lying down, you should look only at the ceiling.
- Keep your neck elongated as an extension of your spine. Do not allow your head to come forward.
- Support your weight firmly on your sacrum and lower back.
- Make your abdomen the point of support and feel it.
- Keep your trunk raised without moving throughout. If you cannot, you may have to work on your abs by doing different exercises before starting on this one.
- Breathing: Inhale at the starting (preparatory) position, exhale at position 2, inhale at
- position 3, exhale at 4, inhale at 5 and exhale as you lower your trunk back down.

How To?

1. Lie on your back with your hands on the back of your head, knees flexed and feet flat on the floor.
2. Raise and lower your trunk, keeping your hips neutral and your elbows open wide.

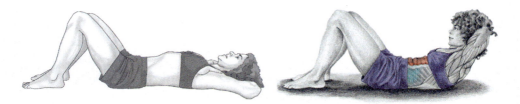

 Notes: There are endless variations of this exercise, including some that affect the original movement, such as oblique ab prep, keeping your trunk raised while moving your arms, combinations involving leg movements, and so on. In ab prep exercises, the elbows must be kept open wide to prevent your lats from engaging to help with the trunk flexion.

Variations: 1. Foam ball between knees

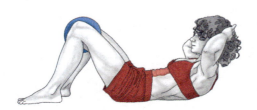

Pressing a ball between your knees works your adductor muscles, adding further benefits to the basic ab prep exercise. You can use this variation provided once you have mastered neutral hips / pelvic stabilization principle.

Adaptations

If your neck hurts, you can do the ab prep exercise at half height using an arc to support your back (see Exercise 3 of Chapter 3, "Adapted Exercises").

You can also place an elastic band along the whole length of your body, pulling with your hands to support your head and neck. This adaptation makes doing the exercise easier (see Exercise 3 of Chapter 3, "Adapted Exercises").

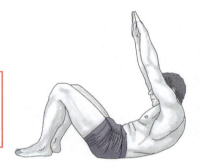

 Common Mistake: Dorsal Hyperkyphosis. Rounding strains the upper back and may occasionally cause chest pain. It is better to raise the trunk less and take all the energy only from the abdomen.

 Common Mistake: Dorsal Hyperlordosis. Your lower back will arch upward if you fail to connect the abdominal transverse muscle, allowing the muscles of the lower back to spring into action. To prevent this, connect the muscles on your front and relax your back. Apply the principle of pelvic stabilization, keeping your hips neutral.

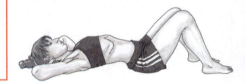

 Muscles Involved

Dynamic Muscles: The rectus abdominis is a spinal flexor and, as such, the main muscle responsible for raising the trunk in abdominal/ab prep exercises. The abdominal obliques share some of the work with the rectus abdominis close the ribcage.

Stabilizing Muscles: The abdominal transverse stabilizes the hips, preventing strain on the lower back.

The lower fibers of the trapezius stabilize the shoulder blades.

Others: The internal and external rotator muscles of the hips keep the legs straight and in line. Main Stretch: Spinal erectors

2 Abdominal — Hundred (3-1)

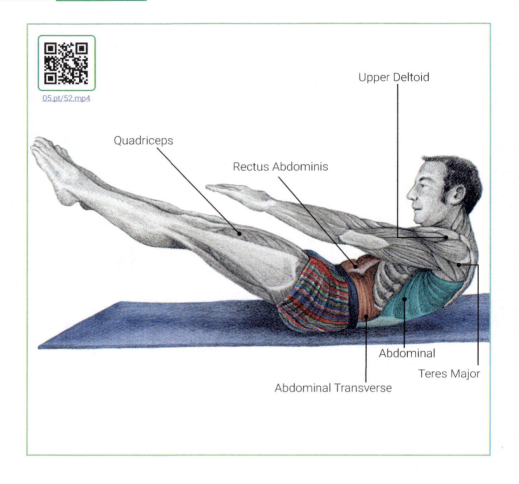

Exercise Benefits and Transfer

- Increased pulmonary ventilation
- Improved aerobic performance
- Increased cellular oxygen exchange.
- Stronger respiratory muscles.

Keys to good form

- Look straight ahead.
- Keep your trunk still as your move your arms.
- Synch the movement of your arms to your breathing, not your breathing to your arms.
- Breathing: Keeping your spine flexed, inhale and exhale in series of five. You can also breathe in and out steadily (for a count of five) instead of taking short, staccato breaths.

How To?

1. Flex your trunk to lift your head, curving your spine in a C-shape. Hold the position.
2. Stretch out your arms and raise your legs higher or lower depending on your abdominal strength. The lower you keep your legs to the floor, the harder it will be to keep your back stable without your lower back arching up off the floor. If this happens, you will need to lift your legs up towards the ceiling.
3. The exercise consists of breathing one hundred times while holding the posture. Position yourself, inhale once only and immediately afterwards exhale five times in short bursts; then inhale five times and exhale another five... and so on until you reach one hundred. Raise and lower your arms following the rhythm of each breath.

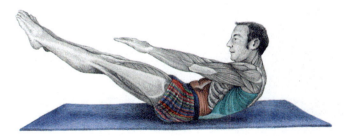

Variations: 1. Seated Hundred:

Sitting cross-legged and your back, complete one hundred breaths while only moving your arms. This exercise is mainly works with the upper deltoids, the teres major and the intercostal muscles.

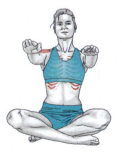

Adaptations

If your abdomen is not strong enough to keep the trunk flexed, you can use an arc to support your back (see Exercise 3 of Chapter 3, "Adapted Exercises").

This is a breathing exercise, so you can do it from a seated position to eliminate the abdominal work (see Variation 1).

 Muscles Involved

Dynamic Muscles: The upper deltoid, latissimus dorsi and teres major move the arms. Since the goal of this exercise is ventilation, the rest of the body should barely move.

Stabilizing Muscles: The muscles that keep the body still in the exercise posture are the rectus abdominis, abdominal obliques, abdominal transverse, quadriceps and psoas. Also the lower fibers of the trapezius, which stabilizes the shoulder blades.

Others: The intercostal muscles work hard, as they are responsible for the movement of the ribcage in lateral breathing, Since this exercise is short and requires little motion, this is barely perceptible from a physical point

 Common Mistake: Lumbar curvature. If you feel your lower back arching upwards because of abdominal weakness, you can correct the posture by raising your legs further to ensure that lumbar region stays flat on the floor. The further you raise your legs, the less the demands on the abdominal muscles.

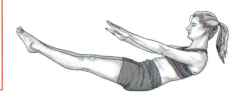

 Notes: You can vary the rhythm of your breathing. Instead of doing the inhalations and exhalations in clusters of five repetitions, you can breathe at a steady pace in five-second intervals. The muscles involved work differently and transference to sports is more oriented towards endurance activities such as long-distance running, in which breathing is deeper than in sprints and middle distance runs.

2. Hundred with Knee

Place yourself in the basic position for doing hundreds, but with your knees flexed. Flex and stretch your knees for every group of five exhalations and inhalations, without moving your arms.

This exercise works the rectus abdominis, abdominal transverse and the quadriceps.

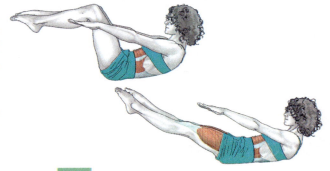

3 | Abdominal | Half roll back (4-1)

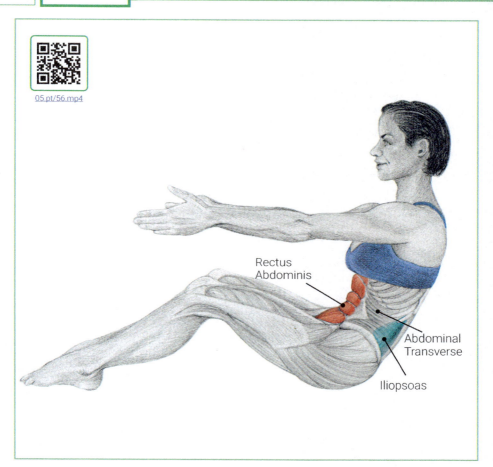

05.pt/56.mp4

Rectus Abdominis
Abdominal Transverse
Iliopsoas

> **Exercise Benefits and Transfer**
>
> - Muscular support for the mechanical stresses to which the lower back region is exposed in everyday life.
> - Support for the midsection of the back by closure of the ribcage.
> - Correct transfer of strength from the hips to the upper and lower body.
> - Muscular and energetic support for movements that you may until now have believed involved only certain parts of the body. For example, if you have to lift a box, your abdomen supports your back and shoulders.

Keys to good form

- Keep your eyes front.
- The ribcage must be kept closed throughout every repetition and series of the exercise..
- Keep your shoulders from hunching forwards, holding them back and away from your ears.
- The first movement requires rounded hips or "retroversion", while maintaining the normal curvature of the rest of the spine.
- Seek an elegant posture for the upper body, maintaining an open chest-shoulder structure.
- Keep your legs hip-width apart and parallel.
- Breathing: Inhale

How To?

1. Sit with arms outstretched and knees flexed.
2. Round and extend your lower back so as to rest your sacrum on the floor.
3. Raise your trunk, undoing the retroversion of your hips until you return to the starting position with neutral hips and a straight spine.

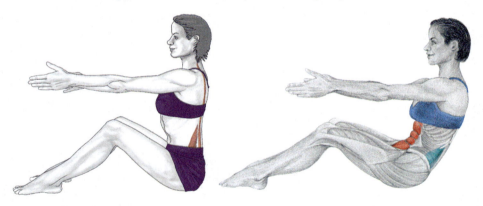

Variations: 1. Tightly Flexed Knees

This is done the same way as the original exercise, but it demands more work from the abdominal transverse muscle. Placing your knees close to your chest enormously increases the intensity of the exercise, and you should therefore only do this variation when you have attained total control of scapular stabilization and lumbar extension (rounding) in the basic half roll back exercise.

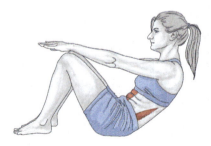

Adaptations

Exercises 3 and 4 of Chapter 3, "Adapted Exercises" will help if you cannot keep your trunk at half height without straining your lower back

 Muscles Involved

Dynamic Muscles: The rectus abdominis and upper fibers of the iliopsoas are responsible for flexo-extension of the lower spine and hips. Stabilizing Muscles: The abdominal transverse handles the strain on the front side of the body so as not to over tax the lower lumbar region. The abdominal obliques are responsible for shutting the ribcage.

Others: The deep back muscles (transverse spinalis and longissimus dorsi, mainly) are in charge of elongating the spine, and the deep hip muscles keep the legs parallel and aligned.

Main Stretch: Spinal erectors.

 Common Mistake: Lumbar hyperlordosis. This consists of letting the lower back arch forward and because the abdominal muscles are not strong enough. Be aware if this happens and correct your posture by rounding your hips further, so as to point the base of your hips (ischia) towards the wall opposite you.

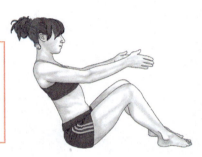

 Common Mistake: Dorsal hyperkyphosis and loss of cervical neutrality. This can happen when you stretch out your arms, as if trying to grab onto something to maintain the half roll back posture. This destabilizes the shoulder blades, placing enormous strain on the trapezius and the spine.

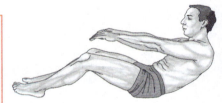

 Notes: Endless variations can be performed by applying small changes to the original pattern of movement, including, for instance, performing an oblique half roll back or holding the posture while rotating the arms. In terms of the biomechanics of the lower spine, a rounding is a form of extension.

This is important given the common misunderstanding of the biomechanics of the hips (also prevalent in relation to the neck), there is a general misunderstanding. Many people think that extending or stretching their hips means sticking their butt out(said in a colloquial fashion) and that stretching or raising their neck means raising your chin up. In fact, the opposite is true in both cases: extending means adopting a rounded posture.

4 Abdominal — Roll up (5-1)

Exercise Benefits and Transfer

- Muscular support to help cope with the mechanical stresses affecting the lower back in everyday life. Support for the midsection of the back by closure of the ribcage. Correct transfer of strength from the hips to the upper and lower body.

- Muscular and energetic support for movements that you may until now have believed involved only certain parts of the body. For example, if you have to lift a box, your abdomen supports your back and shoulders.

- Increase in spinal articulation and articular flexibility.

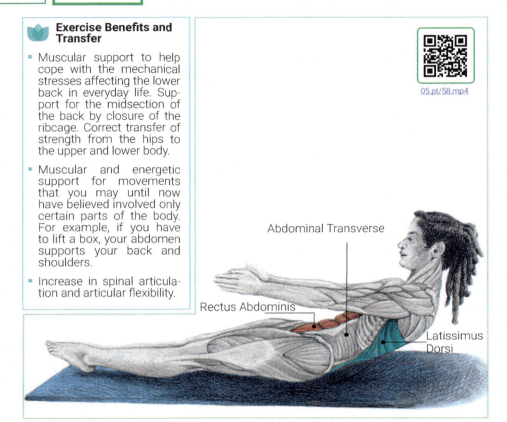

05.pt/58.mp4

Abdominal Transverse
Rectus Abdominis
Latissimus Dorsi

 Note: Just like the half roll up, this exercise is key to doing much of the Pilates method's repertoire efficiently. The right spinal articulation avoids overload in the lumbar and cervical regions, which is the main problem involved in these exercises. Think of a string of pearls and try to ensure there are no unarticulated vertebrae in your spine. Try to visualize how the vertebrae touch the ground in order. Now engage your abdomen to provide the support needed for the movement to flow.

 Muscles Involved

Dynamic Muscles: The rectus abdominis, latissimus dorsi and abdominal transverse work to articulate the spine, ensuring that the movement is sustained and steady. The iliopsoas makes an eccentric contraction during as you lower your torso and a concentric contraction as you lift it.

Stabilizing Muscles: The abdominal obliques stabilize the trunk and close the ribcage, assisted by the shallow and deep muscles of the hips. Others: The scapular stabilizers (mainly the lower fibers of the trapezius) keep the shoulder blades stabilized, and the anterior tibial muscle works to keep the feet straight.

Main Stretch: Spinal erectors.

Keys to good form

- Keep your eyes front so that your gaze matches the movement of your head as it accompanies the torso. You should only be looking directly at the ceiling at the point of lying down.
- Use your arms as levers to help you work against gravity.
- Bring your vertebrae into contact with the ground one by one as if they were a string of pearls. The same during ascent, separating them one by one.
- Begin by raising your head, putting your chin to your neck and keeping your eyes front.
- Breathing: Exhale during descent, inhale while lying down, exhale during ascent and inhale once more while sitting down.

How To?

1. Start from a sitting position, with neutral hips, straight spine, arms outstretched and legs hip-width apart.
2. Articulate your lumbar region, rolling it back until your sacrum touches the ground, and keep going until you are lying down. Engage your abdominal muscles to stop yourself from falling backwards.
3. Raise our trunk beginning at the head and ending with hips, following the same string-of-pearls pattern (see next section).

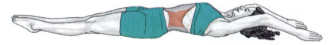

Adaptations

If your abdomen is not strong enough, you can limit the exercise by shortening the descent phase using an arc to reduce the range of movement required (see exercise 3 of Chapter 3, "Adapted Exercises").

You can also use an elastic exercise band to assist your abdomen and remove some of the strain in the lumbar region (see exercise 4 of Chapter 3, "Adapted Exercises").

 Common Mistakes: Pelvic Destabilization: Any imbalance in the strength you exert on the right and left sides of your abdomen will destabilize your trunk and hips You therefore need to ensure that both sides of your hips are equally supported on the ground. The adaptations suggested for this exercise will help you overcome this problem. You should pay special attention to the weaker side.

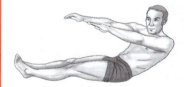

Variations: 1. Oblique Roll Up

Twist your trunk without moving your hips during descent and/or ascent. Imagine that you have a cut under your ribs and a little above the navel. This is where you should twist, maintaining equal support for your hips stay on the floor.

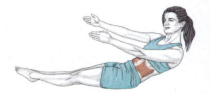

5 Abdominal — Rolling like a ball (8-1)

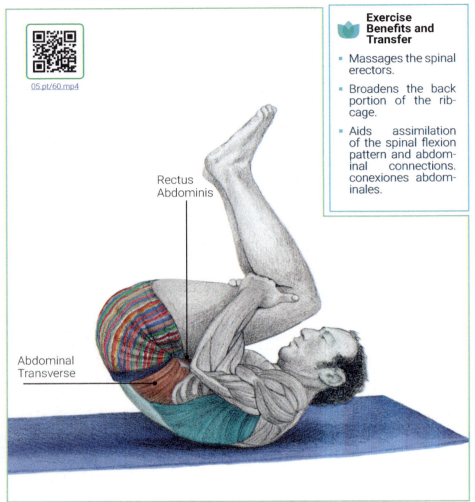

05.pt/60.mp4

Rectus Abdominis

Abdominal Transverse

Exercise Benefits and Transfer

- Massages the spinal erectors.
- Broadens the back portion of the ribcage.
- Aids assimilation of the spinal flexion pattern and abdominal connections. conexiones abdominales.

 Muscles Involved

Dynamic Muscles: None. In this exercise the muscles work in isometric contraction; therefore, there is no movement of body segments or joints. Stabilizing Muscles: Rectus abdominis, abdominal transverse, latissimus dorsi and teres major.

Others: Biceps, triceps and calf muscles work to ensure elegant performance of the exercise and good technique.

Main Stretch: Spinal erectors.

 Notes: Keeping your back rounded may not always be possible, because it depends on your flexibility all along your spine. In such case, do Adaptation 8 (see Annex 1, "Adapted Exercises").

This exercise provides a contact massage on the spinal erector muscles, and although the effects are imperceptible while you do the exercise, you will feel the benefit later.

Keys to good form

- You should pay special attention to the scapular stabilization principle.
- In the elevation stage, lower your gaze to the floor.
- You should feel that your hands are squashed in between your calf muscles and thighs throughout the exercise.
- Keep your eyes open. Structural and muscular imbalances mean that you will tend to stray from the line of rotation line when your gaze is not fixed on a point, especially in this case where the base is unstable.
- Breathing: Inhale while rolling backwards and exhale while rolling forwards.

How To?

1. From a sitting position, flex your knees and grasp the back of your legs behind your knees without linking your hands. Keep your elbows flexed and your shoulders back and away from your ears.

2. Keep your back rounded in both stages of the exercise, which consists of rolling on your back without your head touching the floor in the descent phase or your feet touching it as you return. Your heels should remain close to your glutes throughout, otherwise you will convert the exercise into Variation 2 (Relaxed version).

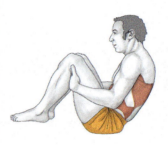

Adaptations

See Exercise 8 of Chapter 3, "Adapted Exercises."

 Common Mistake: Spinal extension in the downward or return phase. If you extend your spine in the descent stage, you will bump uncomfortably against the floor, taking away any benefit from the exercise. Likewise, extending your spine as you come back up may cause strain in the lower back region due to constant flexion and extension of the hips. This exercise therefore requires complete stabilization of the body without flexing the spine in the least.

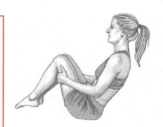

Variations: 1. Ball between the heels and glutes   2. Relaxed Version

Gripping a ball between your calf muscles and hamstrings demands more intense work from your abdominal muscles and activates the hamstrings. This variation is helps with assimilation of the idea of keeping your heels close to the glutes, which may get lost in the effort to roll on your back.

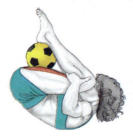

This variant involves doing the exercise without the obligation to keep your heels by your glutes. By allowing you to gain momentum from your legs, this version reduces abdominal workload needed to keep the trunk continuously flexed.

6 Abdominal — One leg stretch (9-1)

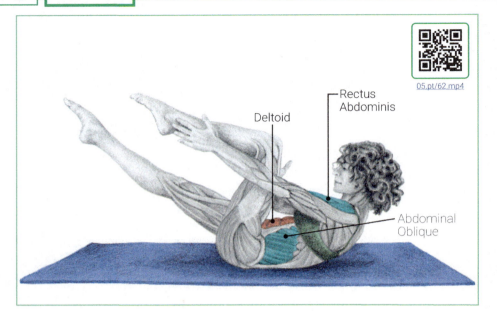

05.pt/62.mp4

Labels: Deltoid; Rectus Abdominis; Abdominal Oblique

 Muscles Involved

Dynamic Muscles: The rectus abdominis is a spinal flexor and is the main muscle responsible for raising the trunk in abdominal exercises. The abdominal obliques assist the rectus abdominis with this work, in particular on the side of the flexed leg.

Stabilizing Muscles: The lower fibers of the trapezius work to stabilize the shoulder blades. This might not seem important at first glance, but the absence of stabilization would result in a hunched back or "dorsal hyperkyphosis" in medical terms (see Common Mistakes).

Others: The internal and external rotator muscles of the hips keep the legs parallel and aligned. Meanwhile, the iliopsoas is responsible for flexing and extending the hips helped by of the navel, technically abdominal transverse muscle. Main Stretch: Spinal flexors, gluteus maximus and posterior deltoid.

 Exercise Benefits and Transfer

- Muscular support to help cope with the mechanical stresses affecting the lower back in everyday life.
- Support for the midsection of the back as a result of closing the ribcage.
- Correct transfer of strength from the hips to the upper and lower body.
- Muscular and energetic support for movements that you may until now have believed involved only certain parts of the body. For example, if you have to lift a box, your abdomen supports your back and shoulders.
- Improved upper-lower body coordination.
- Strengthens cervical muscles.

 Notes: By placing your hands on the back of your neck in exercises involving arm choreography, you can cancel out any arm movements, making it easier to stabilize the shoulder girdle. If your have not yet integrated this principle, one should begin by applying this variation to similar exercises. There will be an intense workload for the abdomen, and once you have gained the necessary abdominal strength, you can bring in the arm movements required.

Keys to good form

- Keep your eyes front, accompanying but not anticipating the movement of your head. You should only be looking at the ceiling when lying on your back.
- Keep your neck elongated as a prolongation of the rest of your spine, and stop your head from moving forward.
- The ribcage must be kept closed throughout every repetition and series of the exercise.
- Do not allow your shoulders to come forward, keeping them back and away from your ears even if you cannot reach your shin and ankle.
- Your hips should not move as you move your legs, and you should feel both glutes resting on the floor with equal pressure.
- Keep your legs parallel and hip-width apart.
- Breathing: Exhale as you raise your trunk and inhale as you lower it.

How To?

1. Lie on your back with your hands behind your neck, knees flexed and feet flat on the floor.

2. Raise your trunk, stretching your hands out towards the shin and ankle of one leg, as shown in the illustration while keeping your knee flexed. Stretch out the other leg while raising it off the floor but without pointing it towards the ceiling.

3. Return to the starting position and raise your trunk once more, switching the position of your arms and legs.

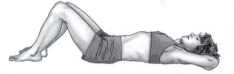

Adaptations

If your neck hurts, you can do this exercise at half height using an arc to support your back. However, this variation means you cannot do the whole exercise, because it eliminates extension of the spine (see exercise 3, Chapter 3, "Adapted Exercises").

 Common Mistake: Dorsal hyperkyphosis. Allowing dorsal rounding overloads the upper back and can cause chest pain. It is better to raise the trunk less far and muster all the energy you need from the abdomen. If you reduce the elevation of your trunk, you will not be able to reach your shin and ankle with your hands. This does not matter initially and can be left as a goal to be achieved later.

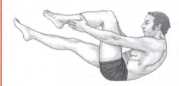

Variations: 1. Hands behind the head

This increases the intensity of the exercise, because it increases the weight on the lever of the upper body. However, it in fact makes it easier to execute, because it eliminates the coordination factor. It also increases the demand on the superficial fibers of the rectus abdominis.

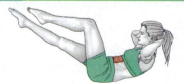

7 Abdominal — One leg stretch oblique (10-1)

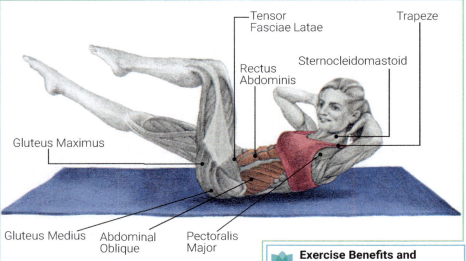

 Muscles Involved

Dynamic Muscles: The rectus abdominis is a spinal flexor and therefore the main muscle responsible for raising the trunk in abdominal exercises, assisted by the abdominal obliques. In this exercise, the muscle on the side of the flexed leg will work harder. Specifically, the working muscles are the oblique minor on the side of the flexed leg and the oblique major on the side of the extended leg.

Stabilizing Muscles: The lower fibers of the trapezius stabilize the shoulder blades. The abdominal transverse muscle holds the pelvis in place.

Others: The internal and external rotator muscles of the hips keep the legs parallel and aligned. Meanwhile, the iliopsoas is responsible for flexing and extending the hips helped by of the navel, technically abdominal transverse muscle.

Main Stretch: Spinal erectors and the quadratis lumborum on the side turned.

 Exercise Benefits and Transfer

- Muscular support to help cope with the mechanical stresses affecting the lower back in everyday life.
- Support for the midsection of the back by closure of the ribcage.
- Correct transfer of strength from the hips to the upper and lower body.
- Muscular and energetic support for movements that you may until now have believed involved only certain parts of the body. For example, if you have to lift a box, your abdomen supports your back and shoulders.
- Increase in upper-lower body co-ordination.
- Strengthens cervical muscles.
- Correct execution of the potentially risky movement of spinal flexion with rotation. Wrongly executed, it can cause vertebral shear and disc herniation.

 Notes: When you are doing oblique abdominal exercises with your hands behind your neck, you should always keep your elbows equally open and motionless in the same position. It is a mistake to put your elbow to your raised knee or, if the knee is not raised, to close your elbow on the side of the trunk that you are raising. This gesture engages the latissimus dorsi to flex the trunk, relieving the abdominals. Also, you should move your head forward so as not to curve your neck too far.

Remember: Your head must rest on your hands and should just hold it but using your arms to help you raise your trunk.

Keys to good form

- Your gaze should accompany the movement of your head and you should avoid looking sideways as you twist your upper body.
- The ribcage must be kept closed throughout every repetition and series of the exercise.
- Your elbows should be more open than closed but not tense.
- Do not try to bring your elbow to your flexed knee. It is better to try to touch your chest to your knee, although you will never reach of course.
- The movement of your legs should not cause movement of the hips. Feel both glutes resting on the floor with equal pressure.
- Keep your legs parallel and hip-width apart.
- Breathing: Exhale as you raise your trunk and inhale as you lower it.

How To?

1. Lie on the floor with your hands behind your neck, knees flexed and feet flat on the floor.
2. Raise your trunk, twisting it towards one of your legs, which should stay flexed while you stretch out and raise the other leg.
3. Return to the starting

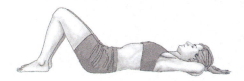

Adaptations

If your neck hurts, you can do this exercise at half height using an arc to support your back (see Exercise 3 of Chapter 3, "Adapted Exercises").

 Common Mistake: Destabilization of Trunk-Hip Structure.

This problem arises when you fail to stretch out your legs completely. When both the upper body and the legs are raised you must keep them balanced: if you do not, one of them will destabilize the support structure. In this case, the legs cause of the support point provided by the hips and lower back.

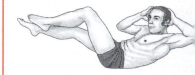

Variations: 1. Ring Between the Knees

This increases the intensity of the exercise, because it also works the adductors. It also helps with execution, however, offering greater pelvic stability.

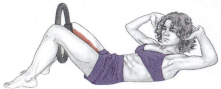

8 Abdominal — Double leg stretch (11-1)

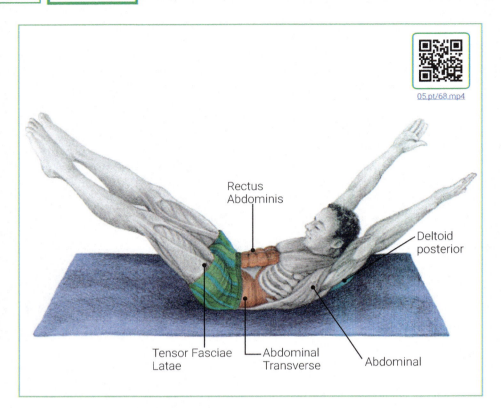

 Exercise Benefits and Transfer

- Muscular support to help cope with the mechanical stresses affecting the lower back in everyday life.
- Support for the midsection of the back by closure of the ribcage.
- Correct transfer of strength from the hips to the upper and lower body.
- Muscular and energetic support for movements that you may until now have believed involved only certain parts of the body. For example, if you have to lift a box, your abdomen supports your back and shoulders.
- Increase in upper-lower body coordination.
- Strengthens cervical muscles.
- Interiorization of the scapular stabilization principle in a difficult situation with transfer to everyday actions involving raised and outstretched arms.

How To?

1. Lie on your back with your arms stretched out behind your head and your hips and knees flexed at 90 degrees.
2. Raise your trunk, bringing your arms forward (you can also do an external rotation of the hip by putting your feet together, separating your knees and bringing both hands to the outside of your legs).
3. Hold the position of your trunk and flex your elbows.
4. Holding your trunk in position, stretch out your knees and raise your arms straight above your head.
5. Flex your knees as you lower your trunk, vertebra by vertebra, keeping your arms straight with your biceps by your ears.

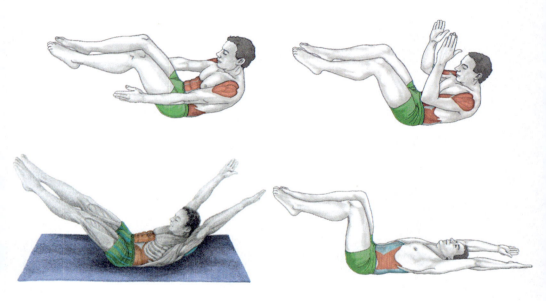

Variations: 1. With Elastic Band

Using an elastic band to provide resistance increases the difficulty of this exercise for the upper body, although it reduces the demand on the abdominal muscles because of the support for the legs.

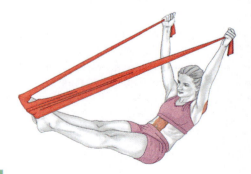

Keys to good form

- Keep your eyes front. You should only be looking to the ceiling when you are lying down flat.
- Keep your neck elongated, as a prolongation of your spine, and try to stop your head from coming forward.
- Support yourself firmly on your sacrum and lower back.
- Feel your abdomen, making it the support point.
- Keep your legs parallel and hip-width apart.
- Breathing: Exhale in position 1, inhale in position 2, exhale in position 3, inhale in position 4.

 Common Mistake: Forward head: Stretching your head forward so that it is no longer in line with your spine will cause tension and strain all of your neck muscles. There is also a point in the cervical spine (neck) that shifts forwards if you do this, causing the intervertebral disc to slide forward, which may put pressure on the nerve root.

Adaptations

If you feel pain in the lumbar region, or even higher up your back, the spinal articulation path can be limited by using an arc to provide support for the back. This prevents the ribcage from opening, so you can do more repetitions without overloading your back (see exercise 3, Chapter 3 "Adapted Exercises").

 Notes: In exercises with broad range of movement, like this one, the use of an elastic band enormously increases the intensity of the exercise. Use a 2 m/6 ft light resistance band. Remember that exercises offer no benefits if the exercise path is not properly executed at all stages.

 Muscles Involved

Dynamic Muscles: The rectus abdominis acts as a spinal flexor and the biceps as elbow flexors in position 2. The coracobrachialis, brachial biceps, pectoralis major, anterior deltoid and subscapular raise the arms in position 3, while the quadriceps straightens the knees. The semitendinosus, semimembranosus, the crural biceps, sartorius, popliteus and the internal and external calf muscles produce flexion of the knee.

Stabilizing Muscles: The lower fibers of the trapezius work to stabilize the shoulder blades. The iliopsoas and transverse abdominal muscle hold the hips in place. The major and minor obliques close the ribcage.

Others: The internal and external rotator muscles of the hips keep the legs parallel and aligned. Meanwhile, the iliopsoas is responsible for flexing and extending the hips helped by connection of the navel (technically the abdominal transverse muscle). Main Stretch: Spinal erectors.

9 Abdominal Scissors (12-1)

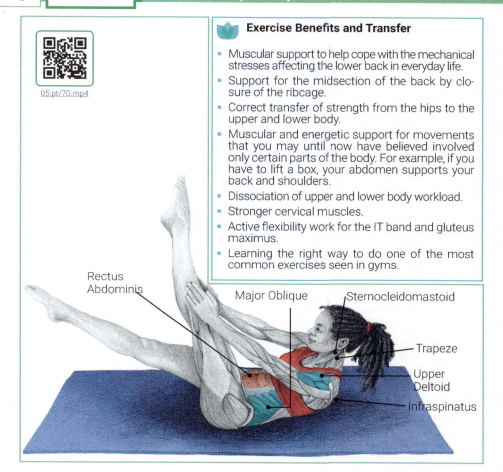

Exercise Benefits and Transfer

- Muscular support to help cope with the mechanical stresses affecting the lower back in everyday life.
- Support for the midsection of the back by closure of the ribcage.
- Correct transfer of strength from the hips to the upper and lower body.
- Muscular and energetic support for movements that you may until now have believed involved only certain parts of the body. For example, if you have to lift a box, your abdomen supports your back and shoulders.
- Dissociation of upper and lower body workload.
- Stronger cervical muscles.
- Active flexibility work for the IT band and gluteus maximus.
- Learning the right way to do one of the most common exercises seen in gyms.

05.pt/70.mp4

Muscles Involved

Dynamic Muscles: The rectus abdominis is the main spinal flexor and, therefore, the main muscle responsible for raising the trunk in abdominal exercises. The abdominal obliques help the rectus abdominis with its workload and are the main muscles in charge of closing the ribcage. In this exercise, the oblique muscle of the leg that is raised towards the trunk works harder.

Stabilizing Muscles: The inferior fibers of the trapezius stabilize the shoulder blades. The anterior deltoid, pectoralis major and coracobrachialis keep the arm raised (antepulsion).

Others: The muscles of the internal and external hip rotators keep the legs parallel and aligned. The abdominal transverse assists when it comes to pelvic stabilization.

Main Stretch: Spinal erectors. IT band and gluteus maximus of the raised leg. Posterior deltoid.

Notes: It is preferable to do smaller and more stable scissors than larger and more unstable ones. The trunk must be kept raised and still during all the scissors repetitions. Since this requires considerable, the exercise is usually done in series of eight repetitions on each leg.

Keys to good form

- Keep your eyes front at all times so that your case follows the movement of your head. You should only be looking at the ceiling while you are lying down.
- Keep your neck elongated as a prolongation of the rest of your spine and do not allow your head to move forward.
- Keep your ribcage closed throughout every repetition and series of the exercise.
- Keep your shoulders from moving forward, holding them back and away from your ears, even if you cannot reach your leg.
- The movement of your legs must not shift the position of your hips and trunk. Try to feel both QL muscles resting against the floor with the same pressure.
- Keep your legs parallel and hip-width apart, and prevent any external rotation of your hips.
- Breathing: inhale as you raise one of your legs towards your trunk and exhale as you raise the other. You can also inhale twice, in staccato, then exhale twice, counting a total of eight breaths on each leg.

How To?

1. Raise your trunk until attaining a good spinal flexion.
2. Raise your legs towards the ceiling and seek the point of balance between the upper and lower body. Your hips and lower back form the fulcrum.
3. Keeping this pose, do "scissors" with your legs but without pulling them up. Use the strength of each leg itself and your abdomen to achieve the movement.
4. You can also do this as a dynamic abdominal exercise by raising and lowering your trunk. To do this, keep legs still while lying on your back and do the scissors as you raise your trunk.

Adaptations

If you cannot keep your trunk raised throughout the exercise, you can also do it at half height using an arc to support your back (see Exercise 3 in Chapter 3, on Adapted Exercises).

In this case, you can also put your forearms on the floor (see Exercise 28 in Chapter 3, on Adapted Exercises).

 Common Mistake: Forward head movement: Allowing your head to come forward causes tension and overloads the neck muscles. There is also a point in the cervical spine that will shift forwards, causing the intervertebral disc to move, which can put pressure on the nerve.

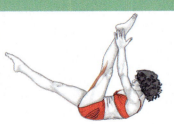

Variations: 1. Hamstring Stretch

This variation works hamstring flexibility by the leg gently towards the raised trunk. The additional stretch obtained increases the distance from the other leg, allowing scissors with a greater range of movement.

10 Abdominal — Half roll back obliques (15-1)

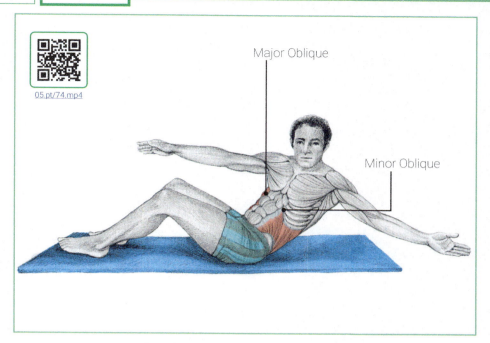

05.pt/74.mp4

Major Oblique
Minor Oblique

Exercise Benefits and Transfer

- Muscular support to help cope with the mechanical stresses affecting the lower back in everyday life.
- Support for the midsection of the back by closure of the ribcage.
- Dissociation of upper and lower body workload.
- Correct transfer of strength from the hips to the upper and lower body.
- Muscular and energetic support for movements that you may until now have believed involved only certain parts of the body. For example, if you have to lift a box, your abdomen supports your back and shoulders.

Keys to good form

- Keep your eyes front throughout the half-roll back and follow your hand with your gaze as you rotate your trunk.
- Keep your ribcage closed throughout every repetition and series of the exercise.
- Stop your shoulders from moving forward, holding them back and away from your ears.
- The first movement rounds the hips while the rest of the spine stays straight, keeping its normal curves. The second movement involves rotation of the trunk just below the rib line.
- Try to combine both movements of the trunk to achieve a smooth flow.
- Seek an elegant posture and an open chest-shoulder structure.
- Keep your legs parallel, hip-width apart. You should feel both of your ischia (the lower part of your hip bone) resting against the floor with equal pressure.
- Breathing: Inhale as you do the half-roll back oblique and exhale as you undo it.

How To?

1. From a sitting position, with arms outstretched forward and flexed knees, round and extend your lower back as in the half-roll back.
2. Rotate your trunk by moving one arm backwards, following your hand with your gaze as you turn.
3. Raise your trunk as your return your arm to the starting point, undoing the rotation.
4. Undo the rounding of

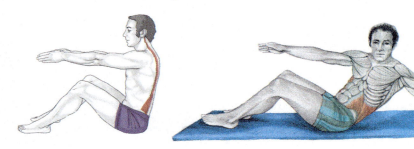

Variations: 1. With Exercise Band

This variant includes upper-body work, specifically involving the teres minor, infraspinatus and posterior deltoid, throughout the external rotation. The superior deltoid and infraspinatus play a role in abduction. Choose a band offering suitable resistance given your physical fitness and mastery of the exercise.

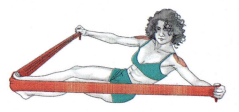

Adaptations

If you cannot keep your trunk at half height without overloading your lower back, Exercise 3 of Chapter 3, "Adapted Exercises", will help

The adaptation in Exercise 4 of Chapter 3 helps perform the half-roll back, but it will intensify the work of the oblique abdominals and upper body, which may be a problem. However, it can be applied if a low-resistance exercise band is used and the movement of the rotating arm is short.

 Muscles Involved

Dynamic Muscles: The rectus abdominis and higher fibers of the iliopsoas are responsible for flexo-extension of the lumbar spine and hips. The abdominal obliques rotate the trunk (oblique minor, towards the side being rotated to; oblique major, in the opposite direction).

Stabilizing Muscles: The abdominal transverse takes the front strain so as not overload the lower lumbar region. The abdominal obliques close the ribcage, playing both a dynamic and a stabilizing role, depending on the muscle fibers concerned.

Others: The deep muscles of the back (transverse spinatus and latissimus dorsi, mainly) are in charge of spinal elongation, while the deep muscles of the hips keep the legs parallel and aligned.

Main Stretch: Spinal erectors.

 Common Mistake: Pelvic Destabilization.

This is caused by failure to dissociate the workloads of the upper and lower body (see "Notes" below).

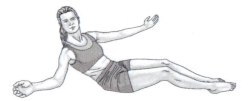

 Notes: In abdominal exercises that include oblique movements, pelvic destabilization and loss of alignment in the legs are frequent. This happens because of failure to dissociate the work of the upper and lower body, which is necessary to keep the lower half of the body still while the upper body moves. To attain dissociation in this exercise, it may be helpful to imagine your body as split in half, like a doll which only can articulate half its body, and, from there, move your trunk without moving your legs in any given position.

2. Hands Behind Neck

More intense exercise for the abdominal muscles, both rectus abdominis and obliques.

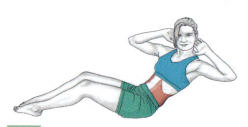

11 Abdominal — Axial Flex (19-1)

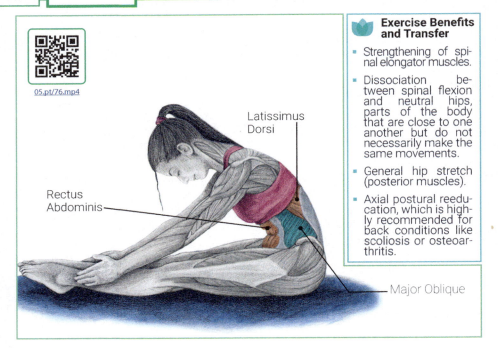

05.pt/76.mp4

Labels: Latissimus Dorsi, Rectus Abdominis, Major Oblique

Exercise Benefits and Transfer

- Strengthening of spinal elongator muscles.
- Dissociation between spinal flexion and neutral hips, parts of the body that are close to one another but do not necessarily make the same movements.
- General hip stretch (posterior muscles).
- Axial postural reeducation, which is highly recommended for back conditions like scoliosis or osteoarthritis.

 Muscles Involved

Dynamic Muscles: Mainly the rectus abdominis in the flexion of the spine, and the lumbar fibers of the iliopsoas. The paravertebral muscles and latissimus dorsi elongate the spine.

Stabilizing Muscles: The abdominal transverse stabilizes the hips, and the abdominal obliques keep the ribcage closed. The lower fibers of the trapezius hold the shoulder blades in place, stabilizing the shoulder girdle. The rectus capitis and longus capitis elongate the cervical spine.

Others: The transverse spinalis help with axial elongation, and the quadriceps in the extension of the knees.

Main Stretch: Spinal erectors, hamstrings and gluteus maximus.

 Notes: This exercise is predominantly abdominal, because the rectus abdominis is the muscle that handles the flexion of the spine. Given the stretch of the whole posterior chain, however, that the stretch will also be felt in the legs if the muscles are tight. This will not be a problem for very flexible people, but poor technique can result in flexion of the hips pushing the legs forwards, which cancels out the abdominal work involved in the exercise.

Variations: 1. Pressing a Ring

Place the ring far enough forward for you to place your hands comfortably on it for support, while keeping your elbows slightly flexed. Push the ring towards the ground while imagining that the strength comes from your abdomen.

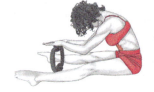

Keys to good form

- Keep your spine elongated throughout the exercise, as if you wanted to increase the distance between one vertebra and the next.
- Keep your hips neutral and stable throughout the exercise. To achieve this, both ischia must stay on the floor.
- The goal is not to bring the trunk down towards the legs but away from them as you flex your spine, resulting the counteraction of opposite forces.
- Breathing: Inhale in the neutral position and exhale as you flex your trunk. Inhale once more as you return to the neutral position

How To?

1. Start from a sitting position, with neutral hips, elongated spine, legs hip-width apart and hands in repose.

2. Flex your trunk while keeping your spine elongated and hips neutral.

3. Extend your trunk once more seeking to maintain the initial postural neutrality of your spine and hips.

Adaptations

If you find it hard to sit with your legs outstretched, you can sit on a cushion to raise the height of the support (see Exercise 7 in Chapter 3, on Adapted Exercises).

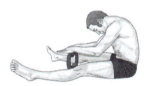

 Common Mistake: Head Forward. This usually happens involuntarily in response to the feeling of a lack of spinal articulation is perceived. You only have to be aware of this mistake to correct it by relaxing your the extensor muscles of your upper back and neck (mainly the trapezius).

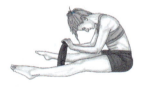

 Common Mistake: Dorsal Hyperkyphosis. Excessive tension in the upper and middle back in order to increase spinal tension. This certainly increases the stretch, but you will be losing the principle of axial elongation and therefore the benefit of the exercise for your joints.

2. Pressing a Ring for Obliques

Press on a ring as in the first variation but with your legs open and one of them inside the ring itself. This will work on the minor oblique on the side of the leg in the ring, and the major oblique on the other side.

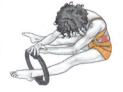

3. Flexing Ankles

This variant increases the stretch in the whole lower body, especially the calf muscles, at the same time strengthening the tibialis anterior (the muscle running down the front of your shin).

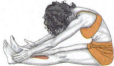

12 Abdominal Seal (21-1)

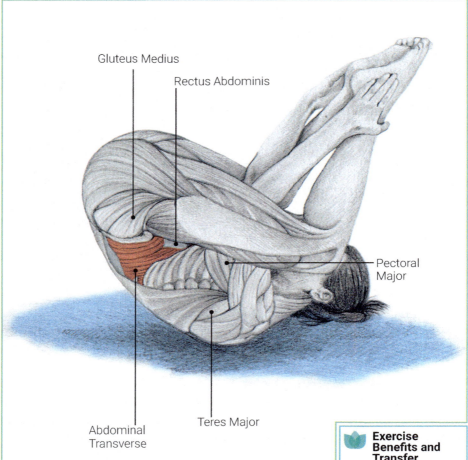

 Muscles Involved

Dynamic Muscles: The sartorius, gluteus medius, gluteus minor and pyramidalis are mainly responsible for adducting the leg, but the effort made by these muscles is barely perceptible because the path of the movements is very small.

Stabilizing Muscles: The rectus abdominis, the abdominal transverse, latissimus dorsi, teres major and upper deltoid.

Others: The biceps and triceps hold the arms together in the clapping gesture.

Main Stretch: Spinal erectors and gluteus maximus and medius.

 Exercise Benefits and Transfer

- Massage on the spinal erectors.
- Expansion of the upper back of the ribcage.
- Assimilation of the spinal flexion pattern, which is closely related to work on the rectus abdominis.
- Fun. This is a good exercise to end a tense Pilates session.

 Notes: This exercise is similar to "Rolling Like a Ball," but far more intense and difficult to perform. Many people simply cannot achieve the initial grip and have to do the variation proposed below. Aside from the unusual grip, this exercise forces you to all the strength in your abdomen to roll onto your back, because you cannot gather momentum with your legs.

Keys to good form

- The "on button" is in the navel and you have to concentrate on this point to generate the momentum for the motion.
- Imagine you are holding a large ball in your arms.
- Keep your eyes open, because structural and muscular imbalances will make you lose your rolling line if you do not keep your gaze fixed on point, especially in this case when your base is so unstable.
- If you cannot clap three times, begin clapping once and increase the number of claps as you improve your motion control from the abdomen.
- Breathing: inhale as you roll backwards and exhale as you roll forwards (rise).

How To?

1. This exercise is similar to "Rolling Like a Ball." Keep your knees apart and feet together. Your arms should go from the outside inwards until your hands are placed on the outside of the feet.

2. Roll onto your back and clap three times with your feet while halting the movement of your body without allowing your head to touch the ground.

3. Roll forwards and clap three times with your feet while halting the movement of your body without allowing your feet to touch the ground.

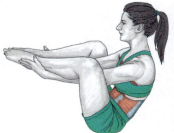

Adaptations

In this case, the adaptation would be to lower the level of the exercise by doing "Rolling Like a Ball" instead until you can improve your control over your abdomen and articulation of the flexed spine.

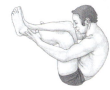

 Common Mistake: Dorsal Hyperkyphosis

Due to the position of the arms, it is usual to raise your shoulders to your ears and "hunch your back." These two gestures are bad for back health and should be avoided. The principles applicable here are scapular stabilization and spinal elongation.

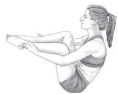

 Common Mistake: Head Forwards

If there is not enough strength in your abdomen or you cannot increase your output further, the common response is to thrust your head forwards to compensate for the lack of movement. This generates significant, potentially harmful strain in the back and neck muscles of the neck.

Variations: 1. Hands on the Outside

The modification consists of placing your arms on the outside of your, rather than from the inside and out. This is recommended in the case of a prominent leg or abdomen, and also if the lower body lacks muscle stability. The muscles working are the same as in the original exercise.

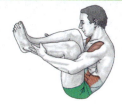

13 Abdominal — Trunk rotation (24-1)

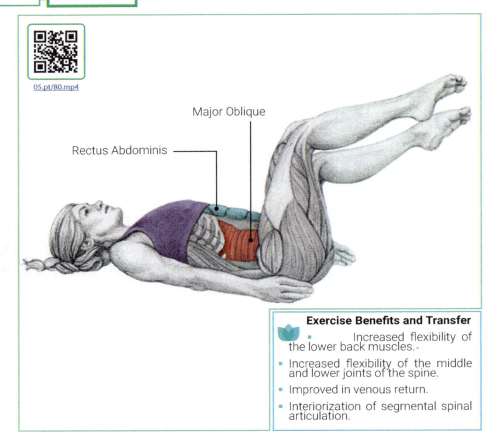

05.pt/80.mp4

Major Oblique
Rectus Abdominis

Exercise Benefits and Transfer

- Increased flexibility of the lower back muscles.
- Increased flexibility of the middle and lower joints of the spine.
- Improved in venous return.
- Interiorization of segmental spinal articulation.

Muscles Involved

Dynamic Muscles: The minor oblique on the side of the rotation and the major oblique on the opposite side act to rotate the trunk.

Stabilizing Muscles: The iliopsoas and transverse abdominal keep the hips in a fixed position.

Others: Rectus abdominis and lower quadratus lumborum (QL).

Main Stretch: QL, intercostals and inferior fibers of the latissimus dorsi on the side opposite the rotation.

Notes: This exercise is recommended to release tension and relax the lumbar region in cases of lower back pain, because it involves a deep knee flex with the thighs held close to the trunk and a reduced range of movements. As a result, it massages the lower sacroiliac fibers and the lower quadratus lumborum.

Keys to good form

- Keep your shoulder and scapula on the side opposite the rotation glued to the floor.
- The obliques do the rotation, but they also close the ribcage, so you must keep them activated from the upper to the lower fibers.
- Try to support yourself as little as possible on your rotation-side arm.
- Do not follow the movement of your legs with your head or turn it in the opposite direction.
- Try to control your energy, performing a slow, deep rotation.
- Breathing: Inhale at the starting position and exhale as you rotate and return your trunk.

How To?

1. Lie on your back with your knees and hips flexed 90 degrees.
2. Rotate your trunk to one side and return to the starting position.
3. Repeat several times on the same side or alternate sides.

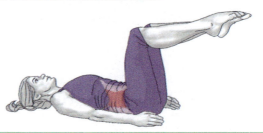

Adaptations

As explained in the "Notes," doing this exercise reduces the intensity of lower back pain considerably.

You can place a cushion under your hips in case of excessive strain on the iliopsoas (see Exercise 6 of Chapter 3, Adapted Exercises).

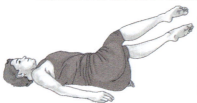

 Common Mistake: Loss of Axial Elongation

Letting your lower back arch creates tension. The solution is to close the ribcage fully and connect the abdominal transverse muscle so as not to lose the abdominal connection present in every exercise.

Variations: 1. With Outstretched Knees

Stretching out the knees involves the quadriceps and increases the activation of the oblique muscles in the abdomen during rotations, because you will be working against a longer lever in the lower body.

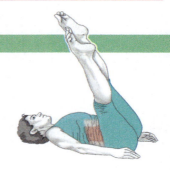

14 Abdominal — Abdominal series (26-1)

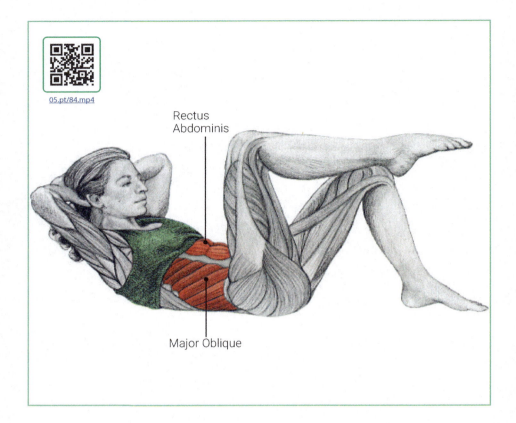

05.pt/84.mp4

Rectus Abdominis

Major Oblique

 Exercise Benefits and Transfer

- Muscular support to help cope with the mechanical stresses affecting the lower back in everyday life.
- Support for the midsection of the back by closure of the ribcage.
- Correct transfer of strength from the hips to the upper and lower body.
- Muscular and energetic support for movements that you may until now have believed involved only certain parts of the body. For example, if you have to lift a box, your abdomen supports your back and shoulders.
- Learning the right way to do one of the most common exercises seen in gyms.
- Improved proprioception of the four abdominal groups.

Keys to good form

- Your gaze should accompany the movement of your head without anticipating it. You should be looking the ceiling only when you are lying down.
- Your head should rest in your hands, which must support but not lift it. Raise your trunk using only the energy generated by your abdominal muscles.
- The ribcage must be kept closed throughout every repetition and series of the exercise.
- Do not allow your shoulders to come forward; keep them back and away from your ears.
- Maintain an elegant posture in your upper trunk and an open chest-shoulder structure.
- Keep your legs parallel and hip-width apart.
- Avoid brusque movements while raising your trunk and raising your leg.
- Breathing: Inhale as you come up and exhale as you go down.

How To?

1. Lie on your back with your knees flexed and your feet planted firmly on the floor.
2. Raise your trunk while bringing your knee up towards your chest, without rotation.

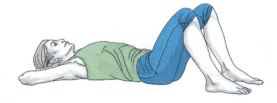
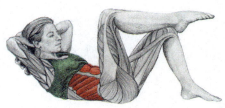

Variations: 1. Basic with Tabletop Legs   2. Oblique with Tabletop Legs

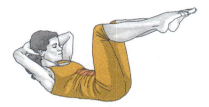
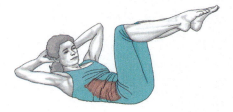

Keep your legs raised and your knees flexed at 90 degrees while you do the abs series. This creates more work for the rectus abdominis and transverse muscles.

Keep your legs raised and your knees flexed at 90 degrees while you do the oblique abs series. This creates more work for the oblique muscles.

Adaptations

If your neck hurts you can do the abs at half height, using an arc to support your back (see Exercise 3 of Chapter 3, Adapted Exercises).

You can also place an exercise band under the whole length of your upper body, using the free end to support your head and neck.

 Muscles Involved

Dynamic Muscles: Rectus abdominis in the flexion of the spine. Oblique minor on the side of the rotation, and oblique major on the opposite side. In the exercises where the hips extend and flex, the workload of the iliopsoas increases (in the original exercise and in Variation 3).

Stabilizing Muscles: The abdominal transverse stabilizes the hips, preventing lower back overload. The lower fibers of the trapezius stabilize the shoulder blades, and the abdominal obliques close the ribcage.

Others: The internal and external hip rotator muscles keep the legs parallel and aligned.

Main Stretch: Spinal erectors.

 Notes: By combining the original exercise with the variations and organizing the whole in alternating series, you can create a very high intensity routine for the abdomen. If you want to do the exercise this way, you should perform series of eight repetitions and rest for a few seconds before tackling the next. This ensures that you will be able maintain good form throughout.

3. One-Leg Stretch

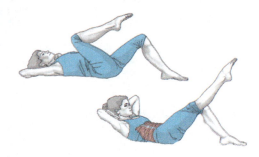

Lying on your back with one knee flexed against your chest, raise your trunk as you stretch the flexed leg out. This works your abdominal transverse muscle and the obliques on the side of the outstretched leg, as well as the quadriceps of the leg raised.

4. Right Angle

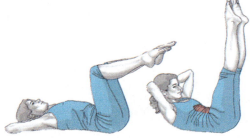

Lying on your back with both knees flexed at 90 degrees, raise your trunk and stretch your legs up towards the ceiling. This increases the workload of all the abdominal muscles, and also engages the quadriceps.

15 | Abdominal | Slow double leg strech) (1-2)

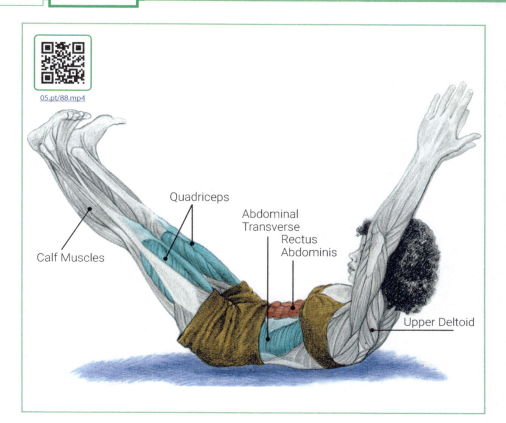

05.pt/88.mp4

 Exercise Benefits and Transfer

- Muscular support to help cope with the mechanical stresses affecting the lower back in everyday life.
- Support for the midsection of the back by closure of the ribcage.
- Correct transfer of strength from the hips to the upper and lower body.
- Muscular and energetic support for movements that you may until now have believed involved only certain parts of the body. For example, if you have to lift a box, your abdomen supports your back and shoulders.
- Increase in upper-lower body coordination.
- Dissociation of the upper and lower body and, within each area, of the arms, knees and hips from the trunk.
- Stronger cervical muscles.
- Interiorization of the principle of scapular stabilization in a difficult position. Transfer to day-to-day actions that require you to hold your hands above your head.

Keys to good form

- Eyes front. You should only be looking at the ceiling when you are lying down.
- Keep your neck elongated as a prolongation of your spine, and do not allow your head to shift too far forward.
- Keep a fixed support on your sacrum and lower back.
- Feel and make your abdomen your support point.
- Keep your trunk raised and motionless throughout. If you cannot, you may need to do further abs work using other exercises before starting on this one.
- Breathing: Inhale in Position 1, exhale in Position 2, inhale in Position 3, exhale in Position 4, inhale in Position 5 and exhale as you come down to rest.

Adaptations

If you feel any pain in your lower back or further up, you can shorten the spinal articulation path using an arc to support your back. This will ensure that your ribcage may open up and will allow you to do more reps than you otherwise could without overloading your back (see Exercise 3 in Chapter 3, Adapted Exercises).

If you feel overload in your neck, place your hands behind your head, which will eliminate the work of the arms from the exercise.

You can also place your forearms on the floor, which will help your abdominal muscles and prevent any risk of injury to your lower back (see Exercise 28 in Chapter 3, Adapted Exercises).

⚠️ **Common Mistake:** Lumbar Hyperlordosis

Whether you work without equipment or use an elastic band, the curvature of your lower back may increase as you raise your arms. This clearly undesirable effect can be corrected by working on your abs.

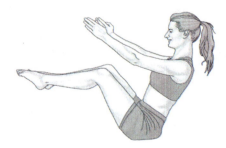

Variations: 1. With an Elastic Band

Working against a resistance elastic band will increase the intensity of this exercise for the upper body, although the support it provides for the legs will reduce the abdominal workload. Choose a long low resistance band for this exercise to allow complete freedom of movement and articular range.

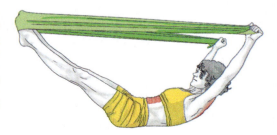

How To?

1. Lie on your back with your hands on the outside of your knees and your hips and knees separated and flexed at 90 degrees (external rotation of the hips).
2. Raise your trunk while flexing your elbows and bringing your knees together as far as the width of your hips.
3. Hold the position of your trunk as you extend your arms and knees.
4. Hold the position of your trunk as you raise your arms and flex your ankles.
5. Lower your arms, until they are parallel to the floor, and straighten your ankles out (plantar flexion).
6. Flex your knees as you lower your trunk, vertebra by vertebra, with your hands on either side of your knees and your knees apart.

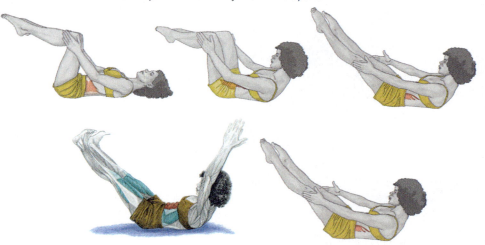

 Notes: In complex exercises, many of the variations and adaptations are designed to eliminate a part of the movement. This removes the workload for some muscle groups and articular structures. The intensity of the exercise decreases, but it is a good way to start without risking injury.

 Muscles Involved

Dynamic Muscles: The rectus abdominis acts as a spinal flexor. The coracobrachialis, pectoralis major, anterior deltoid and subscapularis work to raise the arms in Position 4. The quadriceps extends the knees in Positions 3, 4 and 5. The semitendinosus, semimembranosus, crural biceps, sartorius, gracilis, popliteus and internal and external calf muscles produce the flexion of the knee. There is also work for the external rotators of the hips (pyramidalis, adductors and crural biceps among others).

Stabilizing Muscles: The lower fibers of the trapezius stabilize the shoulder blades. The iliopsoas and transverse abdominal muscles stabilize the hips. The major and minor obliques close the ribcage.

Others: The muscles external and internal hip rotator muscles, keep the legs parallel and aligned. The iliopsoas is mainly responsible for flexing and extending the hips. Abdominal connection (engagement of the abdominal transverse muscle in anatomical terms) helps with this function.

Main Stretch: Spinal erectors.

16 Abdominal — Roll over (3-2)

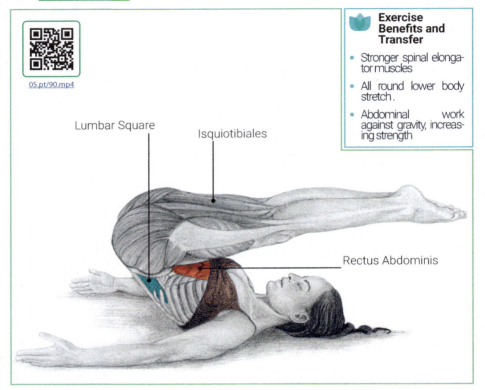

05.pt/90.mp4

Exercise Benefits and Transfer

- Stronger spinal elongator muscles
- All round lower body stretch.
- Abdominal work against gravity, increasing strength

Labels: Lumbar Square, Isquiotibiales, Rectus Abdominis

 Muscles Involved

Dynamic Muscles: Rectus abdominis mainly in spinal flexion, iliopsoas and quadriceps in flexion of the hips and extension of the knees, and paravertebral muscles and longissimus dorsi in spinal elongation.

Stabilizing Muscles: The abdominal transverse works to stabilize the hips, and the abdominal obliques close the ribcage. The lower fibers of the trapezius keep the shoulder blades in place and the shoulders away from the ears. The longus capitis and rectus capitis anterior muscles elongate the cervical spine.

Others: The spinal transverse muscles help with elongation of the spine, and the triceps will be engaged throughout the exercise (although they should not play any major role).

Main Stretch: Spinal erectors.

Variations: 1. Ring Outside the Legs

The exercise is the same except that it increases the muscular workload, especially for the adductors, which must be kept constantly active to stop the ring from falling off.

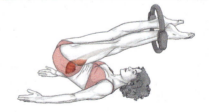

Keys to good form

- Keep all four abdominal groups (rectus abdominis, abdominal transverse and major and minor obliques) working throughout the exercise. Do not use any momentum.
- Stretch your neck, elongating at the back.
- You may use the support of your arms on the floor as long as you keep your shoulder blades stable. With time and as your abs become stronger, you may be able to do this exercise without arm support.
- The final support point should be the upper back, not the neck.
- Breathing: Inhale at the starting position, and exhale as you flex and raise your trunk. Inhale gently when you reach the top and exhale as you extend your spine and descend.

How To?

1. Lie on your back with your arms by your sides and your legs at half height.
2. Flex your trunk slowly and progressively until your legs come back over your head parallel to the floor.
3. Lower your trunk vertebra by vertebra until you return to starting position.

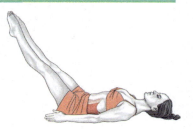

Adaptations

You can do the exercise with your hips raised on a support, which will eliminate the work of the lower back (see Exercise 29 in Chapter 3, Adapted Exercises).

If your lower body chain is too tight or your abdominal muscles are too weak to permit elevation, flex your legs to shorten the lever (see Exercise 20 in Chapter 3, Adapted Exercises).

 Common Mistake: Insufficient Axial Elongation and Scapular Stabilization

This happens when you work from your back instead of from your abdomen. The ribcage opens, the lower back rounds itself, strain increases and the shoulders approach the ears, overloading the upper back and neck.

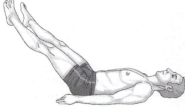

 Notes: The greatest challenge in the roll over exercise is maintaining axial elongation, from hips to neck, throughout the exercise. There is no point in merely raising the trunk without observing the key Pilates principles, and it can be risky. Do not hurry. The spinal articulation work and abdominal strength you achieve from other exercises will eventually make this one easier.

2. Ring between the Legs

Just like in the ring outside variation, this one involves muscle groups that are not worked in the basic the original exercise, in this case the adductors.

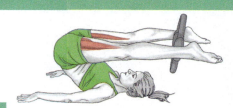

17 Abdominal — Open leg rocker (5-2)

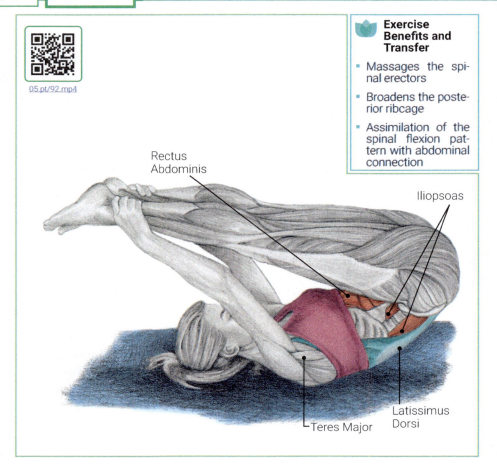

Exercise Benefits and Transfer

- Massages the spinal erectors
- Broadens the posterior ribcage
- Assimilation of the spinal flexion pattern with abdominal connection

Labels: Rectus Abdominis, Iliopsoas, Teres Major, Latissimus Dorsi

05.pt/92.mp4

Muscles Involved

Dynamic Muscles: As hip extensors the hamstrings, and the iliopsoas in eccentric contraction, drive the leg elevation.

Stabilizing Muscles: The rectus abdominis, abdominal transverse, latissimus dorsi, teres major, abdominal obliques and lower fibers of the trapezius maintain scapular and pelvic stability and spinal flexion.

Others: The extensor muscles of the neck keep the head steady, and the lateral fibers of the pectoralis major aid in scapular stabilization.

Main Stretch: Spinal erectors, glutes and hamstrings.

> **Notes:** This is not a difficult exercise to do, but it depends on the flexibility of the posterior chain, so that not everybody can achieve a fluid movement. If you are one, you should opt for another similar exercise, such as the tonic variation of "Rolling Like a Ball", which resembles this one and will allow progression.

Keys to good form

- Pay particular attention to the principle of scapular stabilization.
- You should not feel any momentum during the exercise. Rocking back and forth in this posture should feel natural and easy.
- The key lies in the articulation of the spine, which should be perfectly though not exaggeratedly rounded (which would be a mistake).
- Keep your eyes open, because inherent structural and muscular imbalances in certain postures will tend to make you lose sight of the line of rotation unless you focus on a fixed point. This is especially so in this exercise, where we have such an unstable base.
- Breathing: Inhale as you roll backwards, exhale as you roll forwards.

How To?

1. Grasp your ankles height from a sitting position with knees extended.

2. Keep your spine elongated and gently flexed, as you rock back and forth.

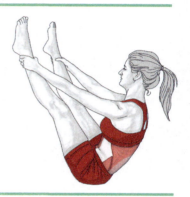

Adaptations

In this case the adaptation consists of flexing the knees, not as much as in "Rolling Like a Ball" but enough to eliminate braking caused by insufficient posterior elongation.

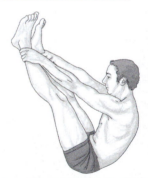

 Common Mistake: Dorsal Hyperkyphosis

When you cannot easily reach your ankles with your hands, because of a tight posterior muscle chain, your shoulder blades can become destabilized resulting in an increased dorsal curve increases. Causing unhealthy kyphosis.

Variations: 1. Flexed Knees Holding the Big Toes

Flexing your knees makes it easier to get into position, but grasping, your big toes makes it more difficult because of the calf stretch resulting from dorsal flexion of the ankles.

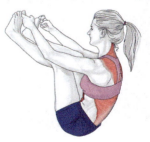

18 Abdominal — Roll up advanced (6-2)

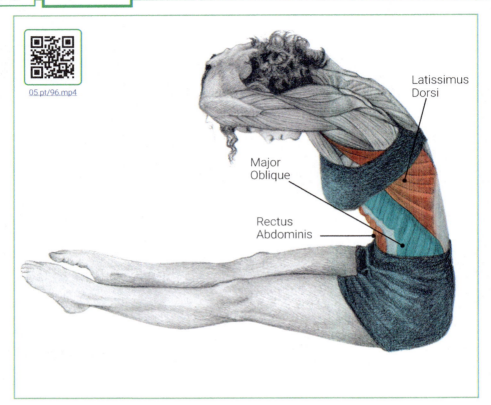

05.pt/96.mp4

Exercise Benefits and Transfer

- Stronger spinal elongator muscles
- Dissociation between spinal flexion and neutral hips. These two body parts are close to one another but there movement is not necessarily the same.
- General posterior chain stretch
- Intense work for the abdominal transverse and iliopsoas.
- Muscle balance in the workload for the latissimus dorsi as a spinal flexor, which act instead of the rectus abdominis, but assists it.

How To?

1. Lie flat on your back with your legs hip-width apart and hands behind your neck.
2. Raise your trunk by flexing your spine, vertebra by vertebra, while keeping it elongated and your legs outstretched
3. Keep on flexing your trunk until you reach attaining the principal position in the Level 1 exercise Axial Flexion, but with your hands behind your neck. You should flex your trunk towards your legs, keeping your hips neutral.
4. Stretch out your spine until you reach the elongated neutral position and lean backwards (gently stretching out your hips).
5. From there, flex your spine and lower your trunk bringing your back to the floor vertebra by vertebra.

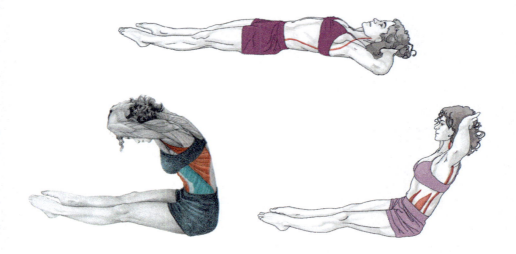

Variations: 1. Twist

Twist your trunk without moving your hips when you are in the sitting position. You can choose whether to do this either before or after flexing your trunk towards your legs, or before extending your spine as you lean back. This variation adds active workload for the abdominal obliques.

Keys to good form

- Keep your spine elongated throughout the exercise, as if you wanted to increase the distance between each vertebra and the next.
- Your hips should be slightly rounded as you raise your trunk. Once you are sitting down and as you lead backwards, you hips are placed in a neutral position. The hips are once again rounded as you lower your back again.
- Flexing your trunk when you are sitting down does not mean flexing the hips. This exercise is not a stretch.
- Keep your elbows more open than closed, but without tension.
- Breathing: Inhale in the supine position, exhale as you flex and raise your trunk. Inhale once more in the sitting position and exhale as you flex your trunk towards your legs. Inhale once more as you extend your spine and hips, and finally exhale as you lower your trunk vertebra by vertebra.

 Common Mistake: Flexing the Hips

Flexing the hips in this exercise would make sense if it were treated as a stretch. However, it is actually a mistake that cancels the dissociation between the neutral hips and moving spine and the work of the rectus abdominis as you flex your trunk towards your legs.

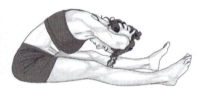

 Muscles Involved

Dynamic Muscles: Rectus abdominis, mainly in spinal flexion, as well as the lumbar fibers of the iliopsoas and the paravertebrals and latissimus dorsi in spinal elongation. The latissimus dorsi also assists spinal flexion if you hold your elbows close to one another. The iliopsoas makes an eccentric contraction during the extension of the hips and as the trunk is leaning backwards.

Stabilizing Muscles: The abdominal transverse stabilizes the hips, while the abdominal obliques keep the ribcage shut. The lower fibers of the trapezius hold the shoulder blades in place.

Others: The spinal transverse muscles help with axial elongation and the quadriceps help stretch out the knees.

Main Stretch: Spinal erectors.

Adaptations

The back can be supported with an arc to eliminate part of the movement to raise and lower the trunk (see Exercise 3 in Chapter 3, Adapted Exercises).

 In other books you may find this exercise listed under the name "Neck Pull." It is classified as a Roll-Up in this book to highlight the similarities between the patterns of movement concerned. Nearly the whole of the neck pull exercise follows the premises of a roll-up in terms of spinal articulation, except for of the part where you lean your trunk back and extend your hips. Hence, the roll-up is the progression exercise towards the neck pull. Raising yourself with your hands behind your head is hard work for the abdominal muscles, though technically correct. This exercise is not so much difficult to do, but very intense.

19 Abdominal — Jack knife (7-2)

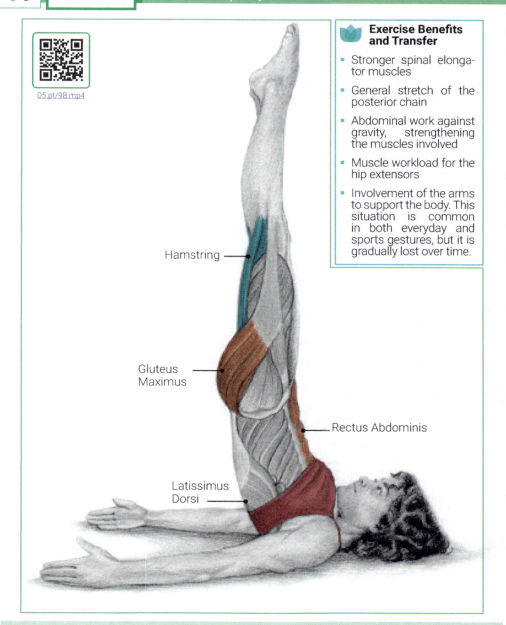

Exercise Benefits and Transfer

- Stronger spinal elongator muscles
- General stretch of the posterior chain
- Abdominal work against gravity, strengthening the muscles involved
- Muscle workload for the hip extensors
- Involvement of the arms to support the body. This situation is common in both everyday and sports gestures, but it is gradually lost over time.

Labels: Hamstring, Gluteus Maximus, Rectus Abdominis, Latissimus Dorsi

05.pt/98.mp4

 Notes: In the Pilates method, inverted supports are held only for short periods: all that is required, in fact, is to adopt the posture and immediately undo it. These exercises involve few repetitions, but they must be fluid and successive, with no moments of rest in between while you are performing the exercise. You need to control momentum and avoid supporting your trunk on your neck for lack of control. Hence the importance of abdominal work alongside the work of the posterior chain, in this case involving your glutes and hamstrings.

Keys to good form

- Keep your four abdominal groups (rectus abdominis, abdominal transverse, major and minor obliques) working actively throughout the exercise.
- Your neck should be elongated and longer at the back.
- Use the support of your arms against the floor. You will feel significant engagement of the triceps.
- The final support should be on the upper back, not on the neck.
- The diagonal inclination of the trunk should be the minimum necessary to avoid using the neck as the final point of support.
- Breathing: Inhale at the starting position, exhale as you flex your trunk and bring your legs back parallel to the floor. Then inhale without changing position and exhale as you raise your legs and torso again. Inhale as you return to the principal roll-over position and exhale as you undo it and return to starting position.

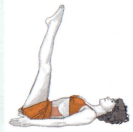

How To?

1. Lie on your back with your arms by your sides and raise your legs towards the ceiling keeping your hips neutral.
2. Flex your spine, vertebra by vertebra, until your legs are parallel to the floor.
3. Extend your spine and hips raising your legs towards the ceiling, aiming to achieve a slightly diagonal position. Support yourself on your upper back and arms.
4. Flex your spine and hips to return to Position 2.
5. Extend your spine, vertebra by vertebra, until you reach starting position with your sacrum on the floor and neutral hips.

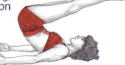

Adaptations

The exercise can be started with the hips already raised to a higher position, so that the lower back work is already done. In this case, you should do very few repetitions because you will not be able to lower your body to the point where your hips are neutral (See Exercise 29 in Chapter 3, Adapted Exercises).

Muscles Involved

Dynamic Muscles: Mainly the rectus abdominis in spinal flexion, and the iliopsoas in flexing the hips; paravertebrals and latissimus dorsi in spinal elongation, and the hamstrings and gluteus maximus in extending the hips during elevation.

Stabilizing Muscles: The abdominal transverse works to stabilize the hips, and the abdominal obliques keep the ribcage closed. The lower fibers of the trapezius keep the shoulder blades in place and the shoulders away from the ears. The longus capitis and anterior rectus capitis act by elongating the cervical spine.

Others: The spinal transverse muscles help with axial elongation, and the triceps work intensely to stabilize the body during elevation and while you hold the final posture.

Main Stretch: Spinal erectors, glutes and hamstrings.

> **Common Mistake:** Cervical Support.
>
> The Pilates method does not use inverted supports on the neck, because axial elongation is lost. In this case, you should not support yourself on your neck even though it would help you maintain stability, because it would cancel out the muscular goal of the exercise.

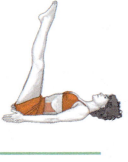

Variations: 1. Flexed Knees

The exercise is done in exactly the same way, but flexing the knees, which reduces the intensity and difficulty of the exercise. Workload is removed from the glutes and hamstrings, and the triceps and abdominal transverse muscles also have less work to do.

20 Abdominal | Teaser (teaser) (9-2)

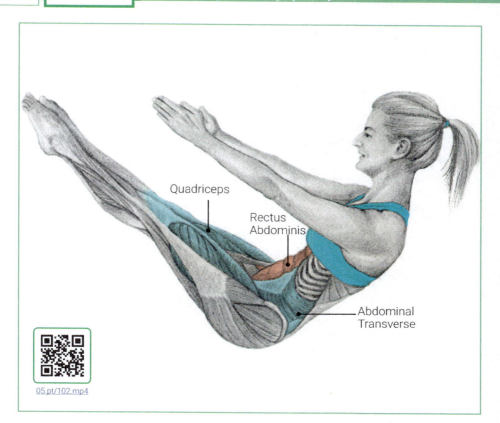

05.pt/102.mp4

Exercise Benefits and Transfer

- General stretch of the posterior chain
- Increase in abdominal strength due to resistance against gravity
- Dissociation between the lower body, which is kept motionless, and the upper body, which is moved.
- Dissociation between the slightly rounded lower back and the elongation of the rest of the spine.

Keys to good form

- Keep your four abdominal groups (rectus abdominis, abdominal transverse, major and minor obliques) working actively throughout the exercise.
- Raise your trunk without momentum, articulating your spine, drawing energy from the abdominal muscles fiber by fiber.
- Keep neck elongated and long at the back.
- As you raise your trunk, imagine also raising your legs even though they do not actually move at all. This image will keep them from falling on the floor.
- Maintain an elegant posture throughout, because you cannot do a good teaser without elongation.
- Breathing: Inhale during moments of less intensity (while lying down and holding the teaser stance) and exhale as you raise and lower your trunk.

How To?

1. Lie on your back with your arms by your sides and your legs diagonally raised to half height.
2. Raise your trunk, from head to hips, while trying not to move your legs. Your arms should stay parallel to your legs. Try to achieve a 90-degree angle between legs and trunk.

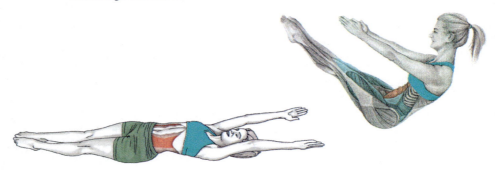

Variations: 1. One Leg

This variation significantly reduces the intensity of the effort required and it can be a good exercise to progressively learn the teaser exercise. The variant is very similar to the original teaser. In muscular terms, the difference is that the major and minor abdominal obliques work harder on the side of the raised leg.

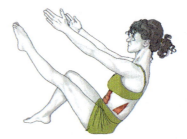

Adaptations

You can do this exercise with your hips raised on a support, which will eliminate the work of the lower back (see Exercise 29 in Chapter 3 on Adapted Exercises).

If your lower body chain is too tight or your abdomen is not strong enough to permit elevation, flex your legs to shorten the lever of the legs (see Exercise 20 in Chapter 3, on Adapted Exercises). Variation 1 also works as an adaptation.

 Muscles Involved

Dynamic Muscles: Mainly the rectus abdominis in spinal flexion, the iliopsoas and abdominal transverse in flexing and extending the hips, and paravertebrals and latissimus dorsi in elongation of the spine.

Stabilizing Muscles: The abdominal obliques keep the ribcage closed. The lower fibers of the trapezius keep the shoulder blades in place and the shoulders away from the ears. The longus capitis and anterior rectus capitis elongate the cervical spine.

Others: The spinal transverse muscles aid in axial elongation, while the quadriceps help to keep the knees outstretched.

Main Stretch: Glutes and hamstrings.

 Common Mistake: Dorsal Hyperkyphosis

This happens when you have to work too hard with your rectus abdominis to flex your spine instead concentrating on spinal elongation. As you hunch your shoulders, your arms will also extend to far, causing scapular instability, which is likely to make your head drop forward.

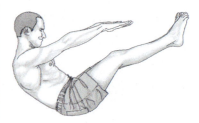

 Notes: You can make the teaser easier to perform by following the right progression, which start with ab prep, half roll back, roll up and the one leg teaser variation. These exercises will warm up your spine, increasing articulation, and prepare your abdominal muscles. This makes it easier to assimilate and integrate the movement required to move the spine.

2. Fit Ball Support

Lying on your back, place your feet on the ball with your knees. Raise your trunk as you stretch out your legs, pushing the fit ball forwards as you rest your feet on it more firmly. The ball will absorb the weight of your lower body, making the exercise easier. These movements must be made simultaneously, otherwise the variation will only make the exercise more difficult.

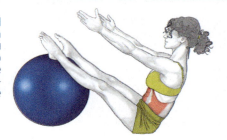

21 **Abdominal** — Hip twist (12-2)

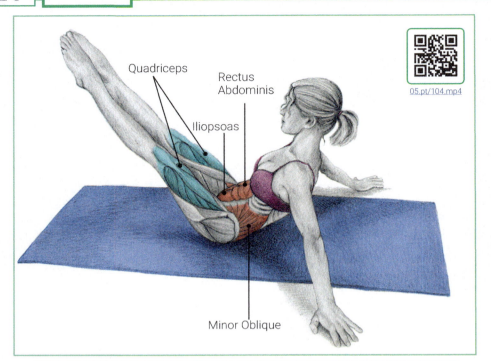

 Exercise Benefits and Transfer

- General stretch of the posterior chain.
- Increased abdominal strength due to resistance against gravity.
- Dissociation between the lower body, which moves, and the static upper body. The whole exercise is powered by the abdomen.
- Dissociation between the slightly rounded lower back and the elongation of the rest of the spine.
- Transfer to movements in which we first sit and only then settle our legs in position, like when you get into a sports car.

 Muscles Involved

Dynamic Muscles: The abdominal obliques work to move the legs from side to side. This effort is shared by the minor oblique on the side of the direction of the leg movement and the major oblique on the opposite side. The paravertebral muscles and longissimus dorsi elongate the spine.

Stabilizing Muscles: The abdominal obliques keep the ribcage shut. The iliopsoas and abdominal transverse maintain the flexion of the hips. The lower fibers of the trapezius stabilize the shoulder blades and keep the shoulders away from the ears. The longus capitis and rectus anterior capitis elongate the cervical spine.

Others: The spinal transverse muscles assist axial elongation, and the quadriceps keep the knees extended. The latissimus dorsi also plays a minor role in the direction of the movement.

Main Stretch: Quadratus lumborum (QL) and abductors opposite the twist.

Keys to good form

- Keep your neck straight and long at the back.
- Imagine a "cut" under your ribs as the point of origin of the lower body movement.
- Use your abdomen to "draw" geometric figures on the far wall projecting through your legs.
- Breathing: You can breathe freely in this exercise. For example, you can inhale for two repetitions and exhale for the next two, or inhale as you twist towards one side and exhale when twist towards the other. If you decide on the second option, you should do the second series of repetitions in the opposite direction.

How To?

1. From a sitting position, lean your trunk backwards, place your hands on the floor for support while slightly flexing your elbows, and raise your legs to form a 90-degree angle with your trunk (teaser position).

2. Move your lower body to the left and right (drawing a half-circle) without allowing any movement of your upper body.

3. Move your legs to draw different patterns, for example figure of eight, squares or circles.

Adaptations

If you cannot manage the elevation because of a tight posterior chain or insufficient abdominal strength, you can shorten the lever formed your legs by simply flexing them. In this case, the adaptation is also a variation.

You can also rest your forearms on the floor for support if you find it difficult to keep your trunk. This will prevent destabilization of the shoulder blades (see Exercise 23 in Chapter 3, Adapted Exercises).

 Common Mistake: Elongation Failure

This happens when the transverse abdominal muscle, abdominal obliques and iliopsoas are not strong enough to handle the workload, so that the rectus abdominis has to take over the work of keeping the spine elevated and flexed. This is the strongest of the abdominal muscles and it is usually activated as a last resort when the others fail. It is better to do shorter series to fix this problem.

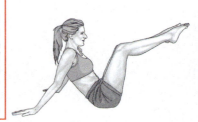

Variations: 1. With Flexed Knees

Shortening the lower body lever considerably reduces the intensity of the exercise. However, flexing the knees increases the difficulty of the exercise, because a new dissociation is added. This variation decreases the workload of nearly all the muscles involved, except for the obliques.

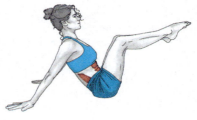

22 Abdominal — Teaser Series (2-3)

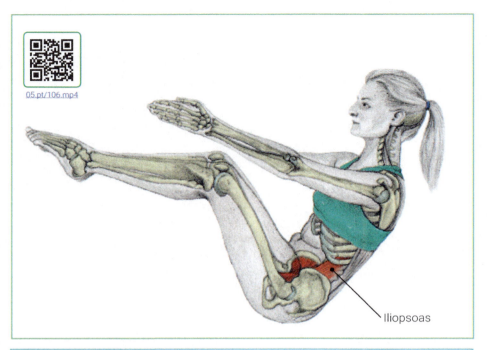

05.pt/106.mp4

Iliopsoas

Exercise Benefits and Transfer

- lGeneral stretch of the posterior chain.
- Increased abdominal strength due to resistance against gravity.
- Dissociation between the lower and upper body.
- Dissociation between the slightly rounded lower back and the elongation of the rest of the spine.
- Dissociation between the rotation of the trunk and stabilization of the hips.

 Notes: Dissociations are necessary and learning them requires time. Think of your body working in parts, some as stabilizers and others in motion. To achieve this, you must try to "restrain" the parts of your body that should remain static, which requires a lot of neuromuscular concentration. It is not for nothing that this an advanced, Level 3 exercise.

Muscles Involved

Dynamic Muscles: Mainly the rectus abdominis to flex the spine, iliopsoas and abdominal transverse to flex and extend the hips, and paravertebrals and longissimus dorsi in the spinal elongation.

Stabilizing Muscles: The abdominal obliques keep the ribcage closed. The lower fibers of the trapezius keep the shoulder blades in place and the shoulders away from the ears. The longus capitis and rectus anterior capitis act to elongate the cervical spine.

Others: The spinal transverses aid in axial elongation and the quadriceps keep the knees extended.

Main Stretch: Glutes and hamstring

Keys to good form

- Keep all four abdominal groups (rectus abdominis, abdominal transverse and major and minor obliques) working actively throughout the exercise.
- Raise your trunk without momentum, articulating your spine, drawing strength fiber by fiber from the abdominal muscles.
- Keep your neck straight and long at the back.
- As you raise your trunk, imagine that you are also raising your legs, even though they do not actually move. This intention will keep your legs from falling to the floor.
- Maintain an elegant movement and posture throughout the exercise: without elongation there cannot be a good teaser.
- Breathing: Inhale in the moments of least intensity (while lying on your back and holding the teaser posture) and exhale as you raise and lower your trunk.

How To?

The Teaser Series is considered an advanced Teaser (Exercise 9 of Level 2 in the Abdominal category), because of the difficulty of maintaining the dissociation between the upper and lower body while one or the other moves. The series are made up of three distinct, separate exercises all done in the teaser position. Each exercise is repeated several times and, if you want, they can be combined to create a high-level exercise chain.

1. Oblique Teaser: Keep your legs and hips still while your rotate your trunk.
2. Hip Teaser: Keep your trunk still while you flex and extend your hips, at all times keeping your knees flexed at a 90-degree angle.
3. Hip and Knees Teaser: Keep your trunk still while you flex and extend your hips and knees, by raising and lowering your knees towards and away from your chest.

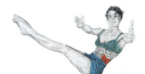 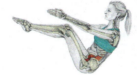 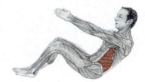

Adaptations

You can start the exercise with your hips elevated on a cushion, which will cut the lumbar workload (see Exercise 29 in Annex 1 on Adapted Exercises).

If your lower body chain is too tight or your abdominal muscles are too weak to permit elevation, flex your legs at least once to shorten the lever (see Variation 1 of the Level 2 Teaser exercise in the Abdominal category).

 Common Mistake: Common Mistake: Pelvic Destabilization

This happens when you fail to dissociate, i.e. when you image that all muscle groups must take part and move in the exercise. This concept of movement falls short in the Pilates method, because some muscles move, others stabilize, others help out and others stretch, and they all do this at the same time.

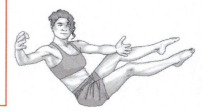

23 Abdominal — Corkscrew (6-3)

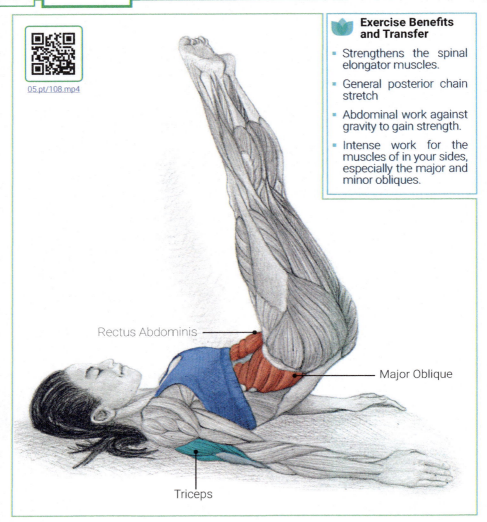

Exercise Benefits and Transfer

- Strengthens the spinal elongator muscles.
- General posterior chain stretch
- Abdominal work against gravity to gain strength.
- Intense work for the muscles of in your sides, especially the major and minor obliques.

05.pt/108.mp4

Muscles Involved

Dynamic Muscles: Mainly the rectus abdominis in spinal flexion, and the abdominal obliques in rotation; iliopsoas and quadriceps to flex the hips and extend the knees; paravertebrals and longissimus dorsi in spinal elongation.

Stabilizing Muscles: The abdominal transverse muscle stabilizes the hips, while the abdominal obliques keep the ribcage closed. The lower fibers of the trapezius keep the shoulder blades in place and the shoulders away from the ears. The longus capitis and rectus capitis anterior elongate the cervical spine.

Others: The spinal transverse muscles help in axial elongation, and the triceps work throughout the exercise although they are not among the main muscles involved.

Main Stretch: Spinal erectors, glutes and hamstrings.

Keys to good form

- Keep all four abdominal groups (rectus abdominis, abdominal transverse and major and minor obliques) working actively throughout the exercise.
- Activate the obliques on one side and then other alternately while you do the trunk rotations.
- If necessary, use your arms to stabilize the position of your body.
- Make the rotation movement "inside yourself," as if you were trapped in a box and had to avoid touching the walls with your legs.
- Keep your neck straight and long at the back.
- You upper back should provide the final support and not your neck.
- Breathing: Inhale in the starting position, and exhale as you flex and raise your trunk. Inhale once gently in the complete flexion position and exhale as you return while doing the rotations.

How To?

1. Lie on your back with your arms by your sides and your legs extended so as to form a pelvic angle of more than 90 degrees.
2. Progressively flex your trunk until your legs are parallel to the floor.
3. Return your trunk to the starting position vertebra by vertebra doing small trunk rotations as you go.

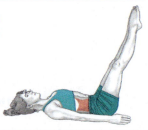

 Notes: "Roll Over" would be a good progression for this exercise, since the form is similar but less intense and complex. Logically, to do a roll over right you also have to make the right progression.

Adaptations

The exercise can be done starting with the hips elevated, which will eliminate the lower back work (see Exercise 29 in Annex 1, Adapted Exercises)

If your lower body chain is too tight or your abdominal muscles are too weak to permit elevation, flex your legs to shorten the lever (see Exercise 20 in Annex 1, Adapted Exercises).

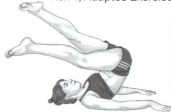

 Common Mistake: Excessive Rotation and Loss of Stability
This happens when your abdominal muscles are insufficiently activated so that you have to draw strength from your back. It can also occur due to excessive momentum and lack of control as you raise your legs and flex your trunk.

Variations: 1. Ring between your Legs

The exercise is done in the same way, but the presence of the ring intensifies the muscle work involved, especially for the adductors. These muscles must be kept constantly active or the ring will fall.

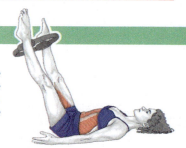

24 Abdominal | Boomerang (9-3)

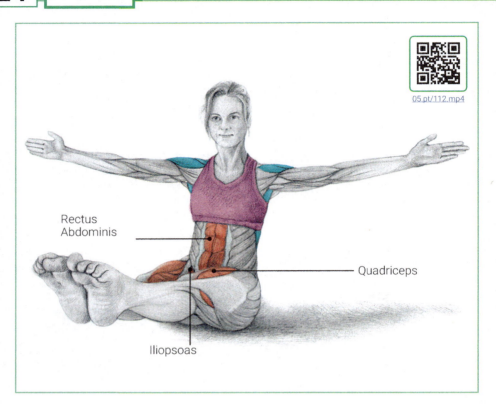

 Exercise Benefits and Transfer

- Strengthens the spinal stabilizer muscles
- General posterior chain stretch Abdominal work against gravity to gain strength.
- Clear example of the principle of integration.
- A challenge for advanced practitioners

How To?

1. Start from a sitting position with outstretched legs, trunk flexed and arms relaxed on either side.
2. Do the descent stage of a roll up and link it to a roll over, ending with your legs parallel to the floor.
3. Undo the roll over and link it to a halfway teaser.
4. Hold the teaser pose while you extend your arms in a cross and "draw" circles with your hands (circumduction).
5. Rest your legs on the floor for support while you close the circle, ending with your arms parallel to the floor and your trunk flexed.

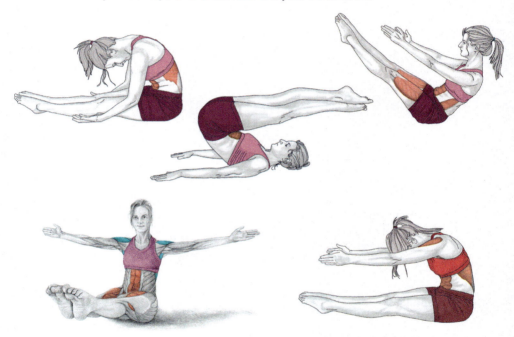

Variations: 1. With Raised Arms

Instead of making circles with your arms you may simply raise them in Position 4. Since this is a simpler gesture, it allows more control over the closure of the ribcage, as well as reducing the time required to hold the teaser position and the overall difficulty of the exercise.

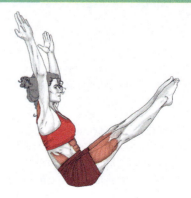

Keys to good form

- Keep all four abdominal groups (rectus abdominis, abdominal transverse and major and minor obliques) working actively throughout the exercise.
- Use the strength of the iliopsoas and abdominal transverse muscles to support the weight of your legs.
- You upper back should provide the final support and not your neck.
- To do this exercise flow right, you need to be able to all of its component parts with good form.
- Breathing: Inhale at the starting position, exhale at the start of Position 2 and inhale once more at the end. Then exhale as you come up into the teaser position, inhale as you perform the arm circumduction and exhale at the end of the exercise.

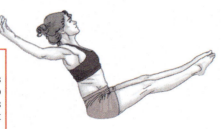

 Common Mistake: Spinal Hyperextension

This happens as you make the circles with your arms if you allow your ribcage to open up. To counteract this effect, which is harmful for your back, you need to connect your abdominal obliques more strongly.

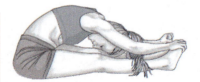

 Common Mistake: Flexing the Hips

At the end of the exercise you need to flex your trunk, not your hips, which should stay neutral throughout the exercise.

Adaptations

All the adaptations described above for the component parts of this exercise flow.

 Notes: Some of the component exercises are described analytically in the explanation of the Boomerang. The trick to performing the exercise successfully is to combine them all in a dynamic, harmonious flow.

Muscles Involved

Dynamic Muscles: The rectus abdominis flexes the trunk. The abdominal transverse and iliopsoas flex and extend the hips. The shoulder muscles intervene in different ways the arm movements.

Stabilizing Muscles: The obliques keep the ribcage closed during the arm circumduction. The quadriceps keep the knees extended.

Others: Quadratus lumborum, latissimus dorsi and pectorals.

Main Stretch: Spinal erectors, lower back, glutes and hamstrings.

1 Mixed — Twist (7-1)

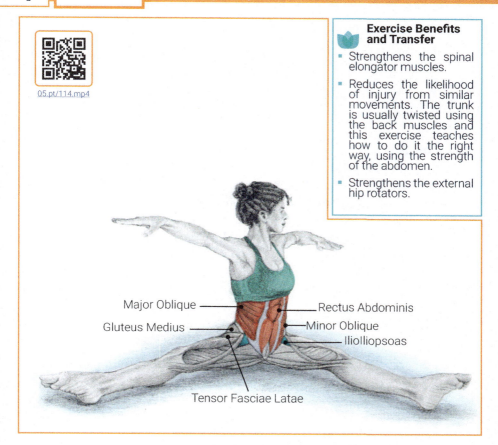

Exercise Benefits and Transfer

- Strengthens the spinal elongator muscles.
- Reduces the likelihood of injury from similar movements. The trunk is usually twisted using the back muscles and this exercise teaches how to do it the right way, using the strength of the abdomen.
- Strengthens the external hip rotators.

05.pt/114.mp4

Labels: Major Oblique, Gluteus Medius, Rectus Abdominis, Minor Oblique, Iliolliopsoas, Tensor Fasciae Latae

 Muscles Involved

Dynamic Muscles: Mostly the major and minor abdominal obliques, which perform the trunk twist. The paravertebrals and longissimus dorsi elongate the spine.

Stabilizing Muscles: The rectus abdominis gives the trunk support, while the abdominal transverse stabilizes the hips. The lower fibers of the trapezius keep the shoulder blades in place, and their action therefore stabilizes the scapular girdle.

Others: The iliolliopsoas, tensor fasciae latae and gluteus medius maintain the stability of the pelvic girdle.

Main Stretch: Quadratus lumborum opposite the twist and hamstrings.

 Notes: If you cannot easily sit with outstretched legs, you can use a cushion, as described in the Adaptations. However, you can flex your knees as much as you need, as long as your hips remain neutral. This is essential for spinal elongation.

Remember that there is no point in doing a twist, or any other exercise, without applying the principles of the Pilates method. In this case, the principles involved are spinal elongation, scapular stabilization and pelvic stabilization.

Keys to good form

- Imagine the crown of your head as growing towards the ceiling.
- To elongate upwards, it is necessary to close the ribcage and connect the navel, as well as imagining the gradual separation of the vertebrae, leaving ever more space between the intervertebral discs.
- Breathing: Inhale as you do the twist and exhale as you return to the center. This breathing pattern will make the exercise easier.

How To?

1. Start from a sitting position, with neutral hips, elongated spine, and arms and legs extended.
2. Twist your trunk, keeping your hips neutral and your arms extended.
3. Undo the twist while maintaining the posture and then twist in the other direction. Your hips must remain neutral and stable throughout the exercise. To achieve this, both ischia must be equally supported on the floor and both legs must be equally extended.

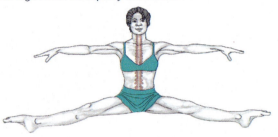

Adaptations

If you find it hard to sit down with outstretched legs, you can raise your support by sitting on a cushion (see Exercise 7 in Chapter 3 on Adapted Exercises)

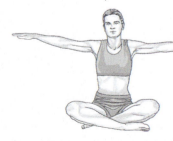

 Common Mistake: Shoulders to Ears

Destabilization of the scapular girdle when you raise your shoulders. This posture overloads the muscles in the back of the neck and upper back, especially the upper fibers of the trapezius.

Variations   1. With an Elastic Band

Sit cross-legged on an exercise band and twist against the resistance of the band. The intensity of the exercise increases the shorter the band is. Do not wrap the band around your hand but rather ball it all up inside your fist, so as not to close of the blood supply. Exhale as you pull against the resistance of the band and inhale in the less intense return stage.

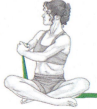 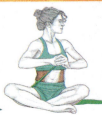

2 Mixed — Saw (14-1)

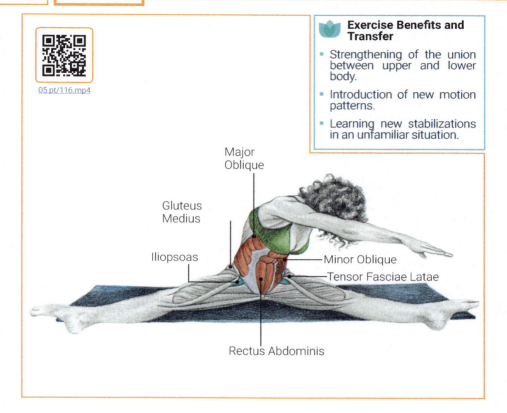

05.pt/116.mp4

Exercise Benefits and Transfer

- Strengthening of the union between upper and lower body.
- Introduction of new motion patterns.
- Learning new stabilizations in an unfamiliar situation.

Labels: Major Oblique, Gluteus Medius, Iliopsoas, Minor Oblique, Tensor Fasciae Latae, Rectus Abdominis

 Muscles Involved

Dynamic Muscles: Mainly the major and minor abdominal obliques, which twist the trunk. Paravertebrals and longissimus dorsi elongate the spine.

Stabilizing Muscles: The rectus abdominis gives the trunk support and the abdominal transverse stabilizes the hips. Gluteus medius and minor, tensor fasciae latae, pyramidalis and sartorius keep the legs apart (abduction). The lower fibers of the trapezius keep the shoulder blades in place; therefore their action is stabilizing the shoulder girdle.

Others: The femoral biceps, pyramidalis and crural square are tasked with external rotation of the hips.

Main Stretch: Lumbar Squareand gluteus maximus on the side opposite the twist. Hamstrings.

 Notes: The saw is as much an exercise for hips, glutes and legs as for the abdomen, because it depends on the elongation of the posterior muscle chains. In sitting exercises, this differentiation is very noticeable. For this reason, and since most people's muscles are very tight in this region, I have decided to include the saw as an exercise for this zone of the body. However, you should bear in mind that the abdominals are the muscles that fallow the trunk to flex and rotate.

Keys to good form

- Grow the crown of your head towards the ceiling.
- To elongate the spine upwards, you need t o close your ribcage and connect your navel, as well as imagining that the vertebrae are being detached from one another, leaving more and more space between the intervertebral discs.
- Your hips must remain neutral and stable throughout the exercise. To make this happen, you need to keep both ischia equally pinned to the floor and both legs equally outstretched.
- Breathing: Inhale from the starting position until you have done the twist, and exhale as you flex your trunk. Inhale once more as you undo the exercise, return to the center and twist in the opposite direction. Exhale as you flex your trunk towards that opposite side.

How To?

1. Start from a sitting position with neutral hips, spine elongated, arms and legs spreadeagled.
2. Twist your trunk, keeping your spine elongated and your arms open in a cross.
3. After the twist, flex your spine while keeping your hips motionless, without flexing them.
4. Undo the flexion and the twist, vertebra by vertebra.
5. Do the same gestures towards the other side, while keeping your spine elongated all the time.

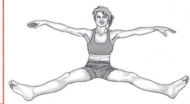

Adaptations

If you find it hard to sit down with outstretched legs, you can raise the point of support by sitting on a cushion (see Exercise 7 in Chapter 3 on Adapted Exercises).

 Common Mistakes: Lack of Axial Elongation and Scapular Destabilization

Destabilization of the scapular girdle due to raising the shoulders, and loss of axial elongation, sinking towards the floor. The former gesture causes overload in the back of the neck and upper back, especially in the upper fibers of the trapezius. The latter gesture causes shear or excessive intervertebral friction during spinal flexion and rotation.

Var iations   1. Flexing the Hip

In this variation, flexing the hips is not a mistake but deliberate. Doing so means work for the hamstrings, glutes and QL during the stretch. This variation makes doing the exercise easier, because keeping your hips neutral as you flex your trunk, as shown in the original exercise, is not a common habit in sports.

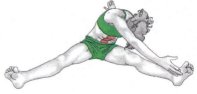

3 | Mixed | Trunk and Legs Lateral Elevation (18-1)

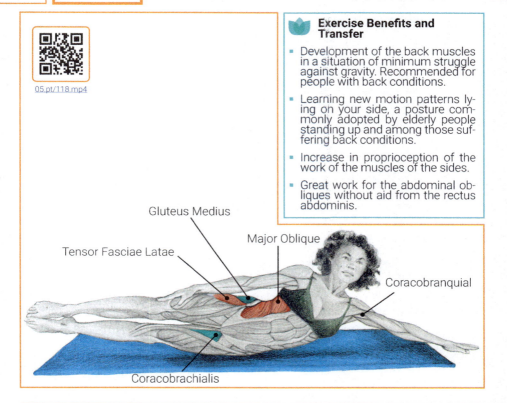

05.pt/118.mp4

Exercise Benefits and Transfer

- Development of the back muscles in a situation of minimum struggle against gravity. Recommended for people with back conditions.
- Learning new motion patterns lying on your side, a posture commonly adopted by elderly people standing up and among those suffering back conditions.
- Increase in proprioception of the work of the muscles of the sides.
- Great work for the abdominal obliques without aid from the rectus abdominis.

Labels: Gluteus Medius, Tensor Fasciae Latae, Major Oblique, Coracobranquial, Coracobrachialis

 Notes: Before taking the plunge into doing this exercise, you need to master the side series of the legs and the side kick variation with arms behind the neck. These two exercises train the strength of the obliques in lateral flexion of the trunk, and the strength of the stabilizing muscles of the shoulder girdle. Otherwise, the trapezius may become overloaded.

 Muscles Involved

Dynamic Muscles: The gluteus medius and tensor fasciae latae abduct the leg. The gluteus medius, gluteus minor and tensor fasciae latae also work to prevent the external rotation that is usually made to draw strength from the quadriceps and iliolliopsoas. Also working are the minor oblique on the side of the raised leg and the major oblique on the opposite side. Finally the anterior tibialis, which makes the ankle flex.

Stabilizing Muscles: The abdominal transverse stabilizes the hips. The trapezius stabilize the shoulder girdle. The spinal extensors avoid the flexion of the trunk as the legs are raised. And the gluteus maximus, along with the hamstrings, keep the hips extended.

Others: The quadriceps of the leg on the floor keeps the knee extended, as the gluteus maximus and hamstrings also keep the side of the hips that rests on the floor extended. The serrates, Coracobrachialisand Pectoralis Majoris, to a lesser degree, keep the stability on the supporting shoulder.

Main Stretch: Lumbar Squareon the side that rests on the floor.

Keys to good form

- Imagine a line drawn from your pinky finger that runs down your side and your leg all the way down to your pinky toe. Support only that line on the ground, "gathering up" everything else.
- Try to extend your whole body and feel it throughout the exercise, without dropping the tonic posture that keeps you supported on your side.
- "Glue" your legs together, from your groin down to your feet, as you raise both legs.
- The trunk barely moves, and the elevation of the legs therefore needs to be very constrained and controlled.
- Your shoulders must be relaxed in order to avoid upper back overload.
- As you raise your legs you must lengthen your neck from behind. Cervical elongation will help in fighting the tendency to flex the spine.
- Breathing: Inhale in the starting position, exhale as you raise one leg, inhale as you join both legs together and exhale as you raise both legs.

How To?

1. Start from a lateral lying position, with arms, trunk and legs completely outstretched and head resting against the arm on the floor.

2. Raise your working leg ten centimeters/six inches more than the breadth of your hips, as you flex your ankle.

3. Lower the leg until it touches the other one, always seeking elongation and muscle tone.

4. Raise both outstretched legs and lower them once more, to start the exercise anew with only one leg.

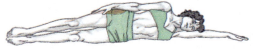

Adaptations

Shorten the lever of your legs by flexing the supporting knee, as shown in Variation 1 of this same exercise (see Exercise 27 in Annex 1 on Adapted Exercises).

You can also flex the knee of the moving leg and even do the exercise with both adaptations.

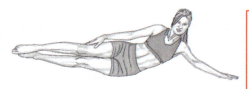

 Common Mistake: Flexing the Hips

A result of lack of strength in the oblique abdominals. When this happens, you tend to draw strength from the quadriceps and iliolliopsoas, which largely nullifies the benefit of the exercise.

Variations   1. Flexed Supporting Knee

This variation reduces the intensity of the exercise, because only one leg is raised. A lower weight of the lever of the legs demands less energy from the obliques. Also, the balance factor is removed because the knee of the lower leg is flexed.

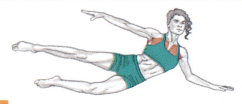

4 — Mixed — Cat and horse (23-1)

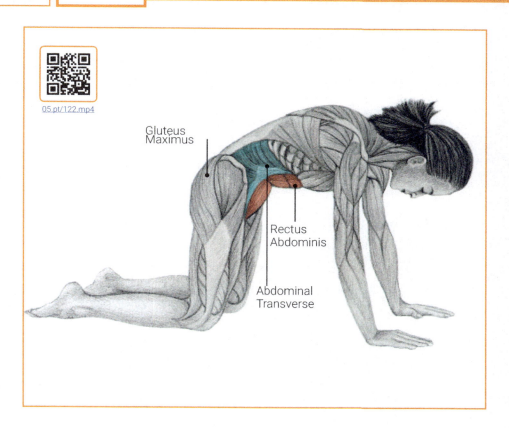

Exercise Benefits and Transfer

- General flexibility of the spine, and particularly of the lower back.
- Scapular stabilization on all fours position.
- Elimination of stress from the back.
- Slight increase in energy; a good exercise to start the day.

Keys to good form

- Keep your lower abdomen (abdominal transverse) active throughout the exercise.
- Don't move your head, which must accompany the movements of your spine.
- Imagine yourself growing towards the ceiling and you will not overload your wrists so much. To do this you must activate all abdominal groups and keep them active throughout the exercise.
- Try to separate your knees and hands from the floor instead of sinking into it.
- Breathing: Inhale during the "horse" stage and exhale during the "cat" stage.

How To?

1. Begin on all fours, with a neutral spine.
2. 2. Flex (arch) your lower back, and by extension all of your spine.
3. 3. Slowly change into an extension (rounding) of the spine.

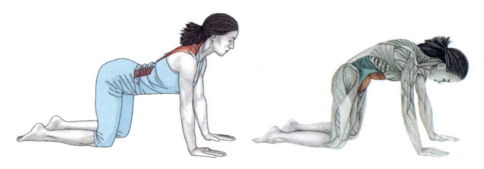

✱ Notes: As a general rule, due to the habit of thrusting the shoulders forwards and overloading the back, it is very easy to round the upper back during the "cat" stage. Therefore you have to try to resist this temptation and pay more attention to rounding the lower back, which in most people requires stretching and articulation.

Variations   1. Superman

From all fours, raise an arm and the opposite leg, elongate these two fully and keep your trunk in place as if you wanted to take off from the floor. This variation adds work for the gluteus of the raised leg and the posterior and superior deltoid of the outstretched arm, as well as the oblique abdominals on the same side.

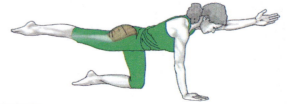

Adaptations

Variation 2 of this exercise is good if you suffer from wrist ache. The forearms can also be placed on the ground for support (see Exercise 25 in Chapter 3, on Adapted Exercises).

 Muscles Involved

Dynamic Muscles: The QL works intensely during the "horse" stage, while the rectus abdominis, the obliques and abdominal transverse work as intensely during the "cat" stage.

Stabilizing Muscles: The abdominal transverse keeps the hips stabilized during the transition from "horse" to "cat." The quadriceps immobilize the knees at a 90-degree angle, and the trapezius keeps the shoulders away from the ears throughout the exercise.

Others: The glutes work as you flex your hips in the "cat" stage.

Main Stretch: In the "cat" stage, spinal erectors, dorsal and lumbar muscles. In the "horse" stage, the Pectoralis Majors gently and, in an eccentric manner, the rectus abdominis.

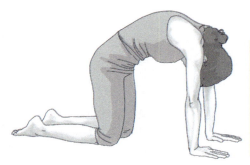

 Common Mistake: Dorsal Hyperkyphosis

When you round your upper back too much, which is easily done due to bad habits, the shoulder blades destabilize and overload is generated in the cervical area and trapezius.

2. Arab Prayer

This variant offers a way to articulate the spine without support from your hands. Turn your body into a rising and falling wave by flexing and extending your knees. Seek an open posture in the "horse" descent and rounding in the "cat" ascent. This variation adds work for the quadriceps.

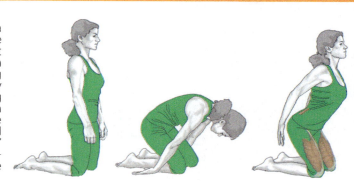

5 — Mixed — Supine squad (25-1)

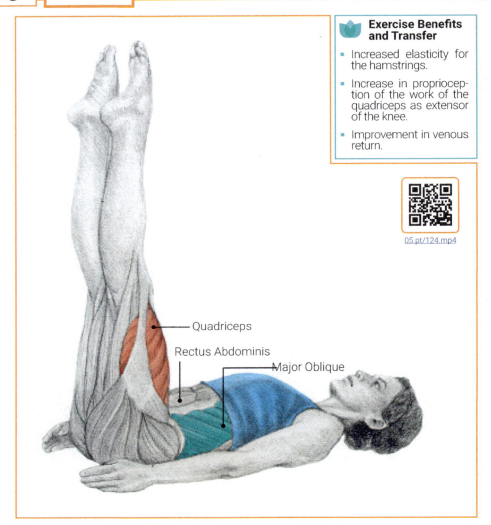

Exercise Benefits and Transfer

- Increased elasticity for the hamstrings.
- Increase in proprioception of the work of the quadriceps as extensor of the knee.
- Improvement in venous return.

05.pt/124.mp4

Labels: Quadriceps, Rectus Abdominis, Major Oblique

Variations

1. Swimming

Do crawl kicks at a steady pace, wider or narrower and at faster or slower speed depending on the series. You will see an increase in the intensity of the exercise for the same muscle groups that work on the original exercise.

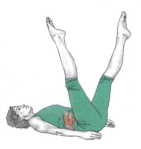

2. Bicycle

Useful to improve the flexibility of the hips. The variant works the same muscles as the original exercise but with different sensations.

Keys to good form

- Extend your knees without blocking them. To achieve this you must think of starting the motion in the quadriceps, not in the joints.
- Keep your thighs motionless and neither too close nor too far from your trunk.
- Imagine and cause the energy to flow from your toes.
- Relax your neck, shoulders and arms.
- Breathing: Inhale as you flex your knees and exhale as you stretch them out.

Notes: If the original exercise is linked with all its variations and the whole is organized as a series of alternating movements, the result will be a combination of high intensity for the legs and abdomen, especially for the abdominal transverse, although this is difficult to feel for most beginners.

How To?

1. Lie on your back with your hips and knees flexed at 90 degrees.
2. Extend your knees completely, then flex them to 90 degrees once more.

Adaptations

A cushion can be placed under the hips in case of excessive tension for the ilioliopsoas or tight hamstrings.

Common Mistake: Loss of Axial Elongation

Letting the lower back arch can strain the back. The solution lies in closing the ribcage well and connecting the transverse. The key is not to lose the abdominal connection that should be present in every exercise.

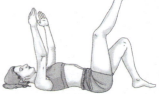

 Muscles Involved

Dynamic Muscles: The quadriceps is responsible for extending the knee.

Stabilizing Muscles: The abdominal obliques keep the ribcage shut. The abdominal transverse and ilioliopsoas fix the hips in a soft lumbar imprint against the floor.

Others: Rectus abdominis and calf muscles.

Main Stretch: Hamstrings.

3. Raising the Hips

Raise your hips a few inches/ centimeters, putting your legs close to your trunk, then undo the rise. This execution means more work for the lower fibers of the abdomen, even though the sensation is general because the rectus abdominis assists the rest of the abdominal muscles.

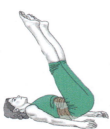

4. Flexing and Extending the Ankles

This involves work for the calf muscles during extension, and of the anterior tibialis in flexing the ankles. The rest of the muscles work exactly like in the original exercise, except the quadriceps, which keeps the knees extended throughout.

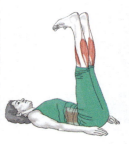

Double leg kick (8-2)

Mixed — 6

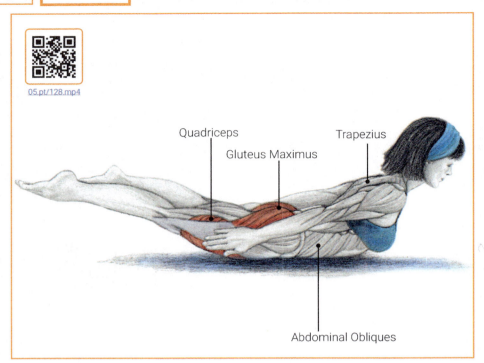

05.pt/128.mp4

Labels: Quadriceps, Gluteus Maximus, Trapezius, Abdominal Obliques

 Exercise Benefits and Transfer

- Strengthening of the elongated lower back.
- Strengthening of the neck muscles towards the left and right (the head is usually turned and supported towards one side).
- Increased elongation of the extended abdominal support.
- External rotation work for the shoulders.

How To?

1. Lie on your front with your elbows flexed, your hands behind your back and your head turned towards one side.
2. Flex your knees to 90 degrees and undo the head turn.
3. Gently raise your trunk, stretch your arms out backwards and lengthen your legs by stretching out your knees.
4. Increase the elevation of the trunk while also raising your legs.

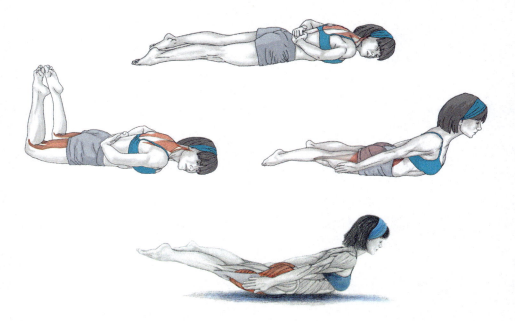

Variations   1. Flexing and Raising Knees in position 4

Raise your legs as you flex your knees in the air, trying to touch your glutes with your heels, not in a kick but in a controlled yet powerful move. This variation increases the workload of the hamstrings.

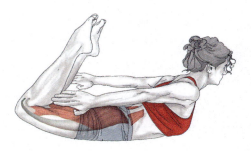

Keys to good form

- Maintain full control as you flex your knees, as if you wanted to push a cushioned surface with your heels and plunge into it.
- The trunk must be raised forwards. Do not raise it towards the ceiling, which would shorten the lower back.
- The legs should be raised backwards, seeking the same elongation as the trunk.
- The closed ribcage and connected core prevent the lower back from curving excessively.
- Breathing: Inhale in position 1, exhale in 2, inhale in 3, exhale in 4, then finally inhale as you return to the starting position. Immediately link to position 2, while respecting the breathing pattern.

Adaptations

If you feel pain in your back or the front of your hips, you may use a cushion for support. This may decrease stability in the exercise, so the cushion must be flat and not too thick (see Exercise 2 in Chapter 3 on Adapted Exercises).

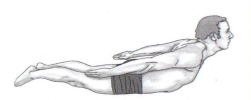

 Common Mistake: Cervical Lordosis and Scapular Destabilization

If you feel that your are failing to raise your trunk, you are likely to compensate involuntarily by raising your head. If you do this, the principle of axial elongation will fail, potentially leading to overload injury to the neck. Raising the chin too far usually causes scapular destabilization.

 Notes: The variation proposed for this exercise may lead to overload in the lower back if not done carefully. It is easier to raise the legs while flexing the knees, therefore, increasing lumbar lordosis without much awareness. The principle of elongation must not be lost. In lumbar work exercises, the structure must always be elongated, separating one vertebra from the other, thanks to visualization and abdominal support.

 Muscles Involved

Dynamic Muscles: The hamstrings and gluteus maximus extend the hips and raise the legs. The lumbar square, spinal erectors and longissimus dorsi are the main muscles in charge of raising the trunk. The splenius and levator scapulae are in charge of turning the head. The rhomboid acts in posterior adduction of the arms and the posterior deltoid in their elevation.

Stabilizing Muscles: The lower fibers of the trapezius keep the shoulder blades stable. The abdominal transverse and obliques restrain excessive elevation of the trunk and support the lower back.

Others: The calf muscles stretch out the ankles (plantar flexion).

Main Stretch: Iliolliopsoas.

7 Mixed — Swimming (10-2)

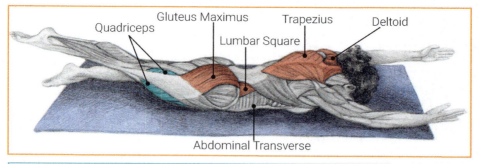

05.pt/130.mp4

Exercise Benefits and Transfer

- Strengthening of the lower back due to the stretch.
- Increase of proprioception of the abdominal work in prone position.
- Especially recommended for correcting postural and functional hyperkyphosis or "hunched back."

Keys to good form

- To raise the leg, Draw strength from your glutes and hamstrings to raise your legs, not from your lower back.
- Imagine the movement as you stretch out your leg as if you wanted to dislocate it from your hips, not as if you were raising it to the ceiling.
- Keep your shoulders retracted as you lift your arm.
- Keep gaze down, looking at the floor throughout, with your head raised as high as your trunk, not more. This will keep your neck neutral and elongated.
- Shoulders, neck and arms must be free from tension.
- Imagine two arrows pulling each leg backwards and a third arrow pulling the trunk forwards. This visualization is important to avoid lower back overload.
- Breathing: Inhale and exhale with each change of arm and leg, or do double breathing.

Muscles Involved

Dynamic Muscles: The muscles of the lower back, gluteus maximus and hamstrings act by extending the hips when the leg is raised. The quadratus lumborum and longissimus dorsi also work, the former increasing the curve of the lower back and the latter elongating the spine. The spinal transverses act extending the spine. The rectus abdominis works in eccentric contraction, giving the elevation support.

Stabilizing Muscles: The lower fibers of the trapezius stabilize the shoulder blades. The abdominal transverse stabilizes the pelvis.

Others: The neck muscles, longus capitis and rectus anterior capitis in particular, elongate the cervical spine.

Main Stretch: Iliolliopsoas and rectus abdominis.

Variations 1. On a Bosu

This variation decreases the stability of the support and therefore the work performed by the abdominal obliques.

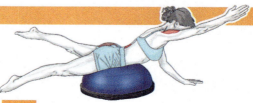

How To?

1. Lie on your front with your hands under your forehead and your elbows open and relaxed.
2. Raise one leg and the opposite arm, stretching them out.
3. Change to the other arm and leg without moving the trunk.

Adaptations

Place a cushion under you between your hips and the lower fibers of the trapezius to avoid flexing and overloading lower back (see Exercise 2 in Chapter 3 on Adapted Exercises).

 Common Mistake: Scapular Destabilization

Scapular stabilization is a basic principle that must be fulfilled in every Pilates exercise. However, it can be difficult to maintain when moving, and especially raising, your arms.

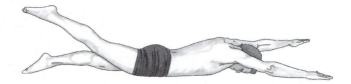

 Notes: The Pilates method does not require you to take in a large quantity of air when breathing. Since the exercises are aerobic, the demand for oxygen is less. Also, in exercises done in a prone lying position with abdominal support like this one, it would be really uncomfortable, apart from technically incorrect. It is already hard enough to keep the ribcage closed and breathe doing Pilates exercises, even those that are done in the most comfortable positions.

8 Mixed — Leg pull front (11-2)

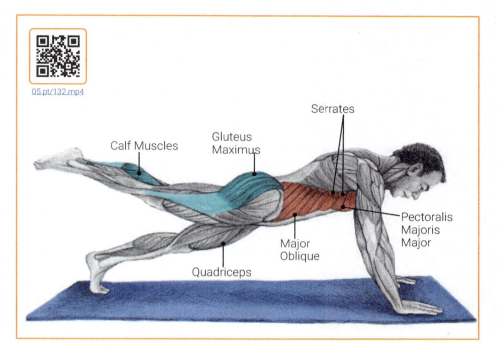

05.pt/132.mp4

 Muscles Involved

Dynamic Muscles: Gluteus maximus, calf muscles and tibialis anterior work to raise and lower the leg.

Stabilizing Muscles: Pectoralis Majoris major, serrates, abdominal transverse and obliques keep the trunk in position. The quadriceps work in keeping the leg outstretched, although you have to take care not to block your knee.

Others: The deep muscles of the trunk aid in stabilizing and keeping the position.

Main Stretch: Iliolliopsoas, calf muscles, plantar fascia and flexors of the wrists.

 Exercise Benefits and Transfer

- Assimilation of the importance of arm support to keep the body in the air. This gesture is less frequent as we grow older and the autonomy of motion decreases enormously.

- Strengthening of the abdomen in a prone position, working against your own weight and gravity.

- Decrease in intra-abdominal pressure against the spine. This kind of abdominal work is recommended for spinal discal conditions. However, exercise needs to be modified in these cases to decrease intensity.

 Notes: Practically the whole body works in a prone position in this exercise. The abdominal work is very intense in this posture, but it will barely be noticed during the exercise. You should include this exercise in your training sessions, even though it is not easy because most of us are unaccustomed to supporting our weight on our hands.

Keys to good form

- Use your abdominals to keep your hips raised. Your abs should feel like a steel plate.
- Tuck your abdomen to stop it from falling, close your ribcage and slightly turn your hips if you feel any pain in your lower back.
- Displace your weight towards the center of your trunk to avoid wrist pain and shoulder overload.
- If your knees hurt, flex them slightly, which will eliminate the blockage. This gesture should not be visible, however.
- Breathing: Inhale while holding the starting position, exhale as you raise your one leg and inhale while you lower it. Maintain the breathing pattern with each kick.

How To?

1. Adopt the plank position, supporting your body on your hands and feet.
2. Raise one of your legs while extending the ankle.
3. Lower your leg, flexing the ankle, and repeat the kick three times, resting your leg on the floor after the third kick.
4. Change to the other leg and repeat.

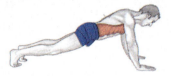 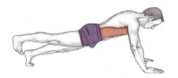

Adaptations

To eliminate the tension that such a long lever implies for the knees and lower back, see Exercise 26 in Chapter 3 on Adapted Exercises.

If your wrists hurt, you may use your forearms for support, although this adaptation increases the workload (see Exercise 25 in Chapter 3 on Adapted Exercises).

 Common Mistake: Pelvic and Scapular Destabilization

Pelvic destabilization occurs when the core muscles of the abdomen are disconnected and the area of the back that matches the disconnect, i.e. the lower back, suffers. As the hips fall to the floor, the shoulders become unstable as well, although this depends on the strength of the serrates, trapezius and latissimus dorsi.

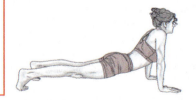

Variations   1. Support on a Box

Resting your forearms on a box (rather than on the floor) will decrease the intensity of the exercise. If you choose this variation, you will have to pay attention to the principle of scapular stabilization, keeping your shoulders retracted. The work of the triceps increases slightly, as long as your body weight is carried backwards.

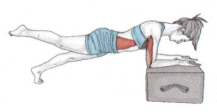

Side bend (13-2)

9 | Mixed

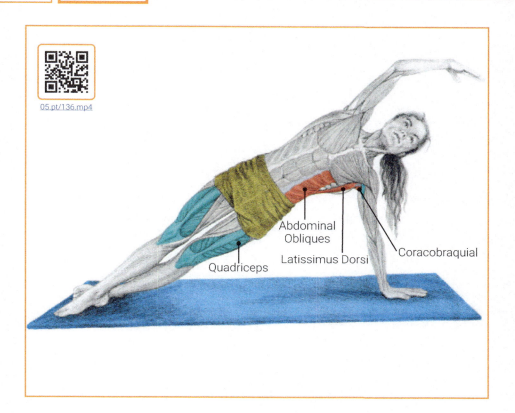

05.pt/136.mp4

Abdominal Obliques
Coracobraquial
Latissimus Dorsi
Quadriceps

Exercise Benefits and Transfer

- Strengthening of the major and minor abdominal obliques.
- Increase of balance in an unusual situation.
- Stretch and strength work for the lateral abdominal chains.
- Global exercise that integrates a great quantity of movements.

Keys to good form

- The initial positional setup is very important for balance in the exercise, so pay attention to step 1 of the next section.
- If you cannot stretch out your knees completely, it may be because your feet are too close to your hips.
- Do the exercise calmly, seeking depth and balance in your movements.
- You can do side bends only in positions 1 and 2, as well as positions 3 and 4.
- Breathing: Inhale during preparation, exhale as you do position 2 and inhale once it is finished. Exhale in position 3, inhale in 4 and exhale as you return to starting position.

How To?

1. Sitting on your side, with your top leg raised and in front and the knee of your bottom leg on the floor. Your feet should be in contact between the heel of the front leg and front of the back foot. Feet, hips and the hand on the floor must all be on the same plane.
2. Raise your trunk by stretching out your legs and bring your arm up and over towards your ear.
3. Turn your trunk inwards and forward, keeping your hips in the frontal plane.
4. Turn your trunk outwards and back, keeping your hips in the frontal plane.
5. Return to position 2, then to 1, then restart the exercise as many times as you please.

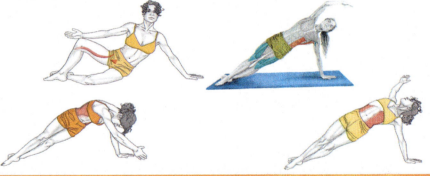

Variations   1. Side Abdominals

Raise and lower your hips supported on your hands and feet, keeping your legs outstretched. This leads to more intense work for the oblique abdominals.

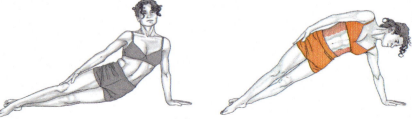

Adaptations

You can use variation 2 as an adaptation if you lack sufficient strength or suffer from wrist or shoulder pain.

If you cannot support your wrist or wish to decrease the intensity of the exercise, you can support yourself on your forearm instead.

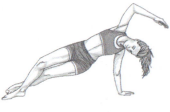

 Common Mistake: Loss of Elongation and Scapular Stabilization

This occurs when you let your shoulder come too close to your ear, i.e. when the effort of scapular stabilization is abandoned. When this occurs it is more difficult to keep your spine elongated, and the side bend appears "weak" without energy.

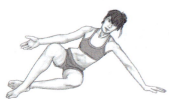

 Common Mistake: Poor Positioning

If your hand and feet are too close to your hips, it will be impossible to stretch out your trunk and legs. This is also the case when your hand or feet are positioned in front of the hips, making it difficult to your keep balance.

 Notes: You should do the combinations that best suit your training goals. In this regard, twists are especially good for working on the obliques. As for positioning, the ideal is to imagine a straight line to sit down on, leaving around 70 cm between the hip and the hand, and between the hips and the feet, even though this reference will obviously depends on your height.

 Muscles Involved

Dynamic Muscles: Abdominal obliques to raise and lower the trunk and in the twists; quadratus lumborum in the twists.

Stabilizing Muscles: Abdominal transverse in stabilizing the hips. Latissimus dorsi, serrates, teres major, trapezius and Pectoralis Majoris major on the supporting side.

Others: Quadriceps in the step from sitting down to outstretched knees. Pyramidalis and sartorius of the raised leg, in keeping the starting position.

Main Stretch: Lateral chain on the raised side.

2. On Knees

Placing your legs together, with flexed knees, decreases the intensity of the exercise enormously and may be a good starting point to tackle side bends for the first time.

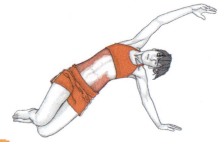

10   Mixed   Push up (14-2)

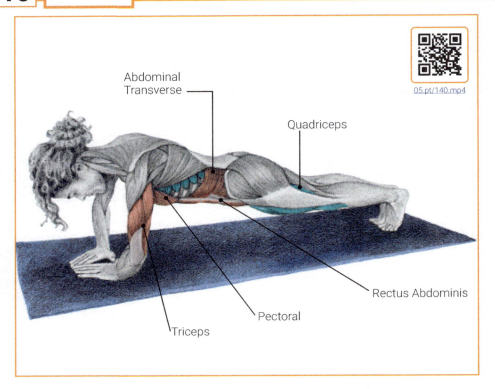

 Exercise Benefits and Transfer

- Correct articulation of the spine as you raise and lower your trunk with outstretched legs.
- Upper body strength.
- Work for the abdominals in prone plank position, which decreases intra-abdominal pressure against the spine. This kind of abdominal work is recommended in the case of spinal discal conditions.

Keys to good form

- Keep your chest close to your legs in order to attain a good flexion of the spine as you lower and raise your trunk.
- In position 1, keep your eyes front, in 2, direct your gaze towards your body, and in 3 and 4, at the floor.
- Engage the strength of your glutes and abdomen to keep the position without fear of lower back overload.
- Keep every muscle in your body engaged so that you feel you are "floating". This will avoid overloading your wrists.
- You should feel your body weight in the abdomen. If it is carried to the upper body, you will place excessive strain on your shoulders and your shoulder blades may be destabilized.
- Breathing: Inhale in position 1, exhale and inhale once more in position 2, exhale in position 3, inhale during flexion and exhale as you outstretch your elbows in Position 4.

How To?

1. Starting from a standing position, flex your spine vertebra by vertebra, until you touch the floor with your hands or come as close as you can.

2. Do a plank. If you need to flex your knees to put your hands on the floor, and walk your hands forward into the plank position, you can do so, but be sure to differentiate the first stage of the exercise from the second.

3. Once you have adopted a good plank position, do three flexo-extensions of the elbows to 90 degrees. Return walking with your hands (about four steps) to position 2.

4. Undo the spinal flexion, vertebra by vertebra until you are standing upright and imagine your self touching the ceiling with the crown of your head.

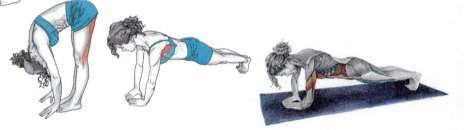

Variations   1. Arabesque

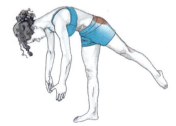

Raise one leg with a slight outer rotation of your hips and keep it raised throughout the exercise. This variation includes work for the gluteus maximus and increases the stabilizing of work of the quadriceps in the supporting leg.

Adaptations

To decrease the tension that such a long lever may create for your knees and lower back, see Exercise 26 in Chapter 3 on Adapted Exercises.

 Common Mistake: Falling Due to Excessive Elbow Flexion

From a biomechanical standpoint, the elbows generate maximum strength at a 90-degree angle. If this angle is surpassed, the overload of effort due to the struggle against gravity and your own weight can make it fail and lead to injury.

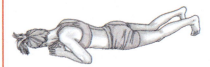

 Common Mistake: Lack of Elongation and Axial Stabilization

Loss of elongation and subsequently of spinal neutrality at any point of the spine will cause overload on the corresponding muscles from behind. For instance, if the abdominal muscles are disconnected, the associated part of the back will suffer.

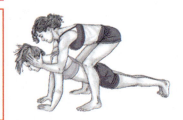

 Notes: This is a mixed exercise that involves work for both the upper body and the abdomen. It is the sum of three exercises the vertical roll-up, the plank and bottoms, each of which is important on its own. As in most Level 3 exercises, you may choose which part of the exercise can be done on its own to work in depth on different goals.

 Muscles Involved

Dynamic Muscles: Rectus abdominis in flexing the trunk. Serrates, pectoralis, rectus abdominis, obliques and abdominal transverses in Position 3. Pectoralis, serrates and triceps in flexing and extending the spine. Hamstrings and glutes in spinal extension to return to starting position.

Stabilizing Muscles: Glutes, quadriceps, abdominals and spinal erectors in Positions 3 and 4.

Others: Latissimus dorsi and rectus anterior capitis major.

Main Stretch: Hamstrings, glutes, Lumbar Squareand calf muscles.

2. Only Vertical Roll

Do only positions 1 and 2. This variation organizes the movement of flexo-extending the spine in a standing position, a very common movement in everyday actions.

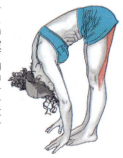

3. Hands Parallel or in Diamond Shape

The hands may be placed in a more or less open diamond shape (the more closed, the more the work done by the triceps and the strain placed on the elbow joints).

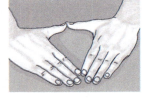

With parallel and separated hands there will be more work for the lateral fibers of the pectorals. The closer your together hands are, the more work for the middle fibers of your pecs.

11 | Mixed | Scissors in air (1-3)

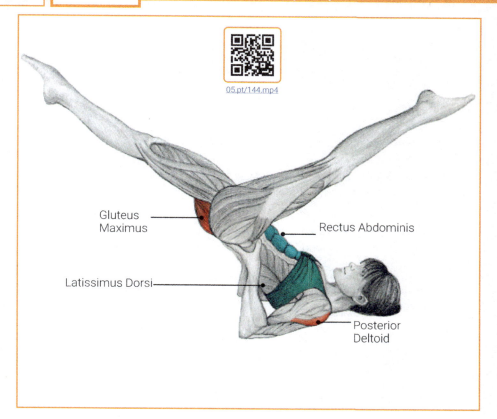

05.pt/144.mp4

Exercise Benefits and Transfer

- Strengthening of the spinal elongator muscles.
- Global stretch of the posterior chain.
- Abdominal work against gravity leading to improved strength
- Muscle work for the hip extensors.
- Involvement of the arms in body support, a common gesture both in everyday life and in sports that is gradually lost overtime.

How To?

1. Lie on your back with your arms by your sides, and legs outstretched and raised to form an obtuse angle (more than 90°) with your and hips, which should be kept neutral.
2. Flex your spine, vertebra by vertebra, to bring legs back over your head until they are parallel to the floor.
3. Extend your spine and hips, raising your legs to the ceiling, aiming for a slight diagonal.
4. Bring one leg towards your and lower the other leg somewhat towards the floor (this movement is similar to the spagat in gymnastics).
5. Return to position 3. Flex your spine and hips to return to position 2.
6. Extend your spine, vertebra by vertebra, to the starting position with your sacrum on the floor and neutral hips.

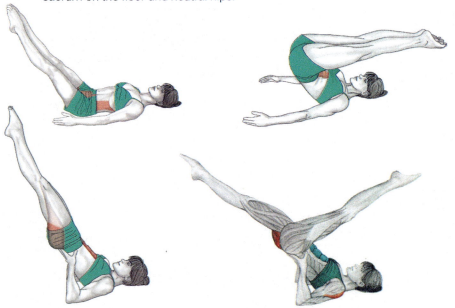

Variations   1. Bicycling in Air

The exercise is similar in positions 1, 2 and 3, and only position 4 is different, when the position of the legs is similar to bicycling. As in the original scissors, your legs should never come close to your face.

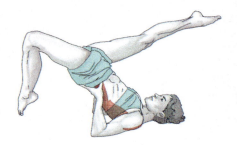

Keys to good form

- Keep all four abdominal groups (rectus abdominis, abdominal transverse, major and minor obliques) working throughout the exercise. Never use momentum in any of its stages.
- The back of your neck must be kept elongated.
- Use the support of your arms against the floor.
- The final support is on the upper back, not on the neck.
- The diagonal inclination of the trunk should be minimal, only as far as necessary to avoid using the neck as the final point of support.
- The scissors should be wide towards the floor and narrow towards the trunk.
- Breathing: Inhale in the starting position and exhale as you flex your trunk and place your legs parallel to the floor.

Adaptations

The exercise can be started with the hips raised, eliminating work for the lower back. In this case, repetitions you should do only a very few repetitions due to the difficulty of lowering the body without reaching the point of neutral hips.

The scissors can also be done using an arc as a steady support for the lower back against an arch (see Exercise 17 in Annex 1 on Adapted Exercises)

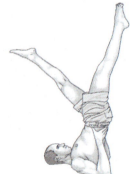

 Common Mistake: Leg to the Face

Keep your legs away from your trunk as you do the scissors, seeking a stretch for the iliolliopsoas of the leg that is closest to the floor.

 Common Mistake: Cervical Support

The Pilates method does not use inverted support on the back of the neck because axial elongation would be lost. In this case, doing so would be a mistake, because it would eliminate all of the muscular goals of the exercise, in spite of helping with stability.

 Notes: Since this exercise is done in air, it is recommended to do a maximum of eight scissors or bicycles per repetition. This guarantees a correct doing of the exercise without tiredness, which could lead to poor technique in what is an advanced exercise.

 Muscles Involved

Dynamic Muscles: Mainly the rectus abdominis in flexing the spine and the iliolliopsoas in flexing the hips; paravertebrals and longissimus dorsi in elongating the spine; hamstrings and gluteus maximus in extending the hips during elevation and especially in the variation Bicycling in Air.

Stabilizing Muscles: The abdominal transverse stabilizes the hips and the abdominal obliques keep the ribcage shut. The lower fibers of the trapezius keep the shoulder blades in place and the shoulders away from the ears. The longus capitis and rectus anterior capitis elongate the cervical spine.

Others: The spinal transverses aid in axial elongation, and the triceps work hard in stabilizing the body during the raising and keeping of the final pose.

Main Stretch: Iliolliopsoas of the leg approaching the floor; glutes and hamstrings of the leg approaching the trunk.

12 Mixed — Swan dive (3-3)

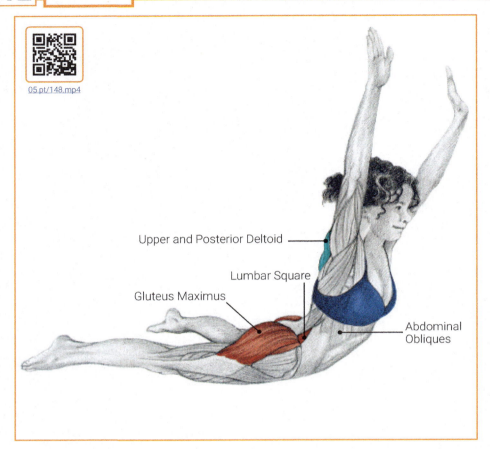

05.pt/148.mp4

 Exercise Benefits and Transfer

- Strengthening of the posterior and support for the anterior muscle chain.
- Introduction of new motion patterns.
- Learning new stabilizations in an unusual posture.
- Ability to react and dissociate the trunk and arms.

Keys to good form

- Keep your glutes, legs, and all of your back muscles steady and engaged.
- Imagine yourself as a seesaw rocking on your upper body.
- Do not look at anything, so as to keep your neck under control and the maintain inertia of the rocking movement.
- Breathing: Inhale in the starting position, exhale as you rock forwards, inhale as you rock backwards and exhale when you stop.

How To?

1. Lie face down on the floor and raise your trunk supporting yourself on your flexed hands and elbows (without touching the floor).
2. Extend your arms forwards and upwards, keeping your trunk elongated and your spine extended.
3. Holding this arc with your body, raise your legs without using your arms for support.
4. Lower your legs again until they touch the floor and end the exercise by putting your hands on the floor again as in position 1.

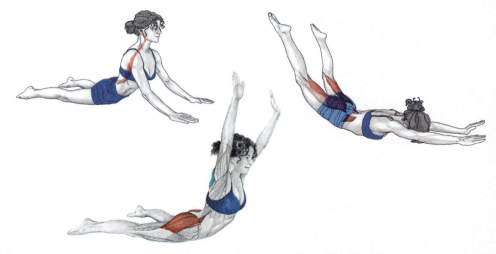

Variations   1. With Forearm Support

In this variant, it is not the hands that are placed on the floor for support but the forearms, keeping, your triceps more relaxed. This reduces the level of the exercise.

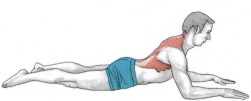

Adaptations

You can shorten the lever formed by your arms by putting your hands on your forehead. This will eliminate the feeling that your face is about to hit the ground (see Exercise 2 in Annex 1 on Adapted Exercises).

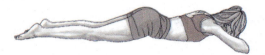

 Common Mistake: Flexed Hips During Rocking
This happens when you cannot keep both body halves elongated, and also in response to unaccustomed, slightly intimidating posture and movement.

 Notes: A lot of repetitions in this exercise involves a significant workload for the lower back, it is therefore not advisable to do long series. The complexity of Level 3 exercises requires care, attention and meticulous correction of your technique. They might be fun and challenging, but to succeed and enjoy them you have to practice and assimilate previous knowledge.

 Muscles Involved

Dynamic Muscles: The anterior deltoid raises the arms at the start of the exercise.

Stabilizing Muscles: Rhomboids, trapezius and spinal erectors keep the trunk elongated and the shoulder blades stabilized. The deltoid works by keeping the arm raised and steady as your rock back and forth. Connection of the abdominal transverse muscle protects the lower back. The lumbar muscles, along with the glutes and quadriceps, keep the lower body boat-shaped.

Others: The longissimus and rectus anterior capitis elongate the cervical spine. The triceps work for a short time while your arms resting on the floor. Main

Stretch: Anterior muscle chain.

2. Steady Rocking

Try to link two or three rocking movements together. To do this variation right you need good stabilization control of the whole posterior muscle chain.

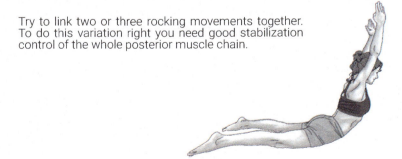

13   Mixed   Leg pull (4-3)

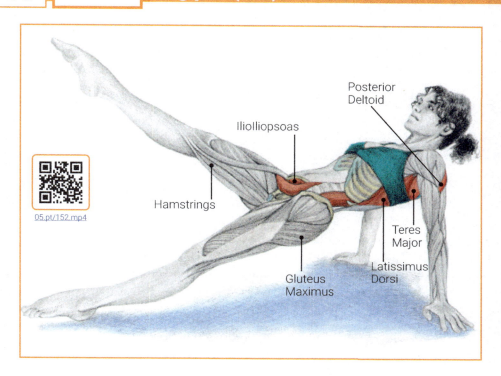

05.pt/152.mp4

Exercise Benefits and Transfer

- Strengthening of the union between upper and lower body.
- Introduction of new motion patterns.
- Learning new stabilizations in an unusual situation.

Keys to good form

- Make sure your shoulders, trunk, hips and legs form a straight line.
- Turn your abdomen into a wooden plank.
- Round your hips a little so that you do not forget about them.
- Raise your legs as much as can while keeping your hips your neutral but no more.
- Breathing. Inhale in position 1, exhale as you raise your leg, inhale as you lower your leg, exhale while raising the other leg, and so for as many repetitions as you please

How To?

1. Support your body face up on your hands and feet to form a plank and look at the ceiling.
2. Raise one leg while extending the ankle. Bring this raised leg towards your trunk while keeping your hips neutral.
3. Lower the raised leg while flexing the ankle, until you put your foot on the floor.
4. Change to the other leg and repeat.

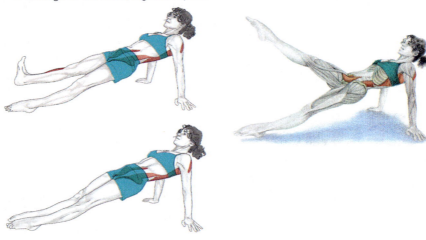

Variations 1. With Forearm Support and Flexing your Ankle as you Flex your Hips

You can increase the intensity of the exercise with these two moves. If you flex your ankle as you bring your hips towards your trunk you will increase the stretch for the hamstrings, while supporting your trunk on your forearms reduces the "in-the-air" component of the exercise. This has the effect of limiting the number of muscles that can aid in stabilizing your trunk, making scapular stabilization more difficult.

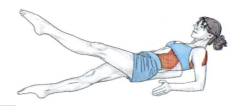

Adaptations

Shorten the lever of your legs by flexing the supporting knee, as described in Variation 2 of this exercise (see Exercise 27 in Annex 1 on Adapted Exercises).

You can also flex the knee of the moving leg, or even do both adaptations at the same time.

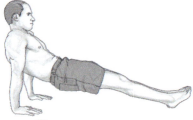

 Common Mistake: Scapular Destabilization
This happens if you allow your shoulders to come too close to your ears, because you cannot keep the lever of your trunk in the air.

 Muscles Involved

Dynamic Muscles: The iliolliopsoas flexes the hips and the leg approaching the trunk. The abdominal obliques on the same side aid in the same action.

Stabilizing Muscles: In the external rotation of the shoulders, infraspinosus, teres minor and posterior deltoid; in retropulsion, posterior deltoid, latissimus dorsi and teres major; in stabilizing the hips, abdominal transverse and glutes; in extending the knee, quadriceps; in flexing and extending the ankle, anterior tibialis and calf muscles.

Others: The whole body partakes isometrically in keeping this pose.

Main Stretch: Hamstrings.

 Notes: We humans are more able to withstand gravity in prone aerial poses than in supine aerial poses, and we are anyway more used to the former position than to the latter. In this exercise you should pay special attention to scapular and pelvic stabilization, and to pressure on the knees.

2. Flexed Supporting Knee

You can reduce the intensity of the exercise with this variation, which limits the length of the lever formed by your legs. This is a good option for painful or hypermobile knees.

14 — Mixed — Control balance (5-3)

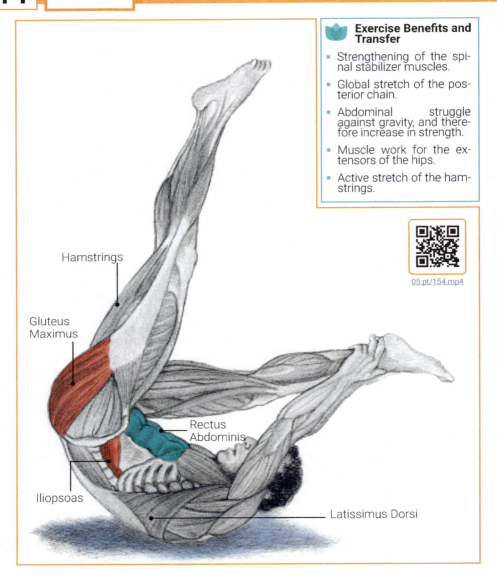

Exercise Benefits and Transfer

- Strengthening of the spinal stabilizer muscles.
- Global stretch of the posterior chain.
- Abdominal struggle against gravity, and therefore increase in strength.
- Muscle work for the extensors of the hips.
- Active stretch of the hamstrings.

05.pt/154.mp4

Muscles Involved

Dynamic Muscles: Mainly the rectus abdominis in flexing the spine; the iliopsoas in flexing the hips; paravertebrals and longissimus dorsi in elongating the spine.

Stabilizing Muscles: The abdominal transverse works stabilizing the hips and the abdominal obliques keep the ribcage shut. The longus capitis and rectus anterior capitis muscles elongate the cervical spine.

Others: The spinal transverses aid in axial elongation, while the latissimus dorsi and pectoralis partake in approaching the trunk with the leg.

Main Stretch: Hamstrings and gluteus maximus.

Keys to good form

- Keep all four abdominal groups (rectus abdominis, abdominal transverse, major and minor obliques) working throughout the exercise. Never use momentum at any stage.
- The back of your neck must be kept elongated.
- The final support rests on your upper back, not on your neck.
- The diagonal inclination of the trunk should be minimal and only as necessary so as not to use the neck as the final support point.
- The scissors should open wide towards the floor but be narrow towards the trunk.
- Breathing. Inhale in the starting position, exhale as you flex your trunk and place your legs parallel to the floor. Inhale and exhale again in that stance. Inhale on your way to position 3 and subsequently draw complete breaths to the rhythm of the movement of your legs.

 Notes: The starting and final position of this exercise imply significant activation of the abdominal transverse, which is necessary not to overload the lower back. The iliopsoas also works more. Meanwhile, not relying on your arms for support increases the difficulty considerably in comparison to similar exercises such as Scissors in Air or the Jackknife.

How To?

1. Lie face up with your arms extended behind your, your legs at an angle above 90 degrees and neutral hips.
2. Flex your spine, vertebra by vertebra, until your legs are parallel to the floor.
3. Extend your spine and hips to raise your legs towards the ceiling, seeking a slight diagonal.
4. Bring one leg towards your trunk while the other stays at a diagonal pointing towards the ceiling. Repeat with the other leg.
5. Return to position 3, then flex your spine and hips to return to position 2.
6. Extend your spine, vertebra by vertebra, until you return to the starting position, with your sacrum resting on the floor and neutral hips.

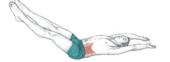 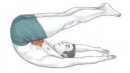 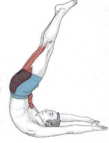

Adaptations

You may start the exercise with your hips already raised using an arc, which will eliminate the workload of the lower back. Take care not to hit the arc as you lower your legs (see Exercise 29 in Annex 1 on Adapted Exercises).

You can also do the scissors with continuous support for the lower back on the arch (see Exercise 17 in Annex 1 on Adapted Exercises).

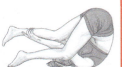 **Common Mistake:** Loss of Aerial Posture

This occurs when the kick is excessive or because your muscles are not strong enough to hold the position. In this case, do as many adaptations as you need until you improve these two aspects. You can also begin with similar but less complex exercises.

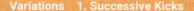

Variations   1. Successive Kicks

You can do as many kicks as you wish, as long as you maintain correct technique. This increases the difficulty of the exercise because you will be keeping your body in the air for longer.

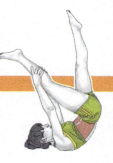

15 — Mixed — *Side kick kneeling (7-3)*

Exercise Benefits and Transfer

- Development of the scapular stabilizer muscles in a situation of intense effort against gravity.
- Learning new motion patterns in an aerial lateral position.
- Increased proprioception of the work of the muscles in your sides.
- Learning new patterns for pelvic stabilization and muscle balance between the upper and lower body.

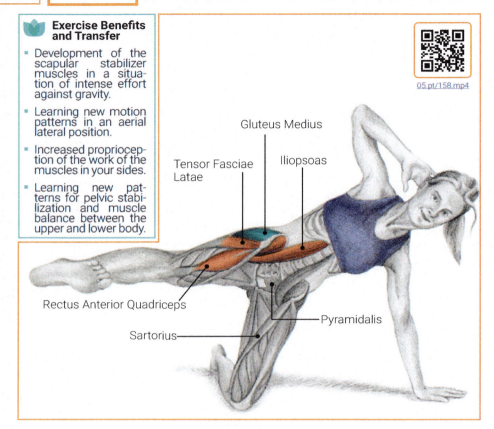

05.pt/158.mp4

Labels: Gluteus Medius, Tensor Fasciae Latae, Iliopsoas, Rectus Anterior Quadriceps, Sartorius, Pyramidalis

Keys to good form

- Imagine that your body is caught between two walls to avoid pushing your hips backwards and allowing your chest to sink towards the floor when you do the exercise.
- Stick your butt out as you kick (anteversion and not retroversion of the hips in anteversion) to compensate for any possible flexion.
- Imagine you are trying to kick your leg over a fence.
- Try to stretch out your whole body and feel its tension throughout the exercise, without leaving the engaged posture that is keeping the muscles of your lower side active.
- If you cannot keep your hand behind your head, place it on your forehead.
- Breathing: Inhale in the neutral position, exhale during the forward kick, inhale as you return to the starting position and exhale during the back kick.

How To?

1. Kneel in an upright position, flex your trunk to the side and put your hand in the floor, on the same plane as your knee.
2. Raise your working leg as high as your hips and do a forwards kick with a flexed ankle, keeping your hips neutral and your spine elongated.
3. Take your leg to the starting point, extending your ankle.
4. Do a back kick and return to the starting position. Realiza otra patada hacia atrás y vuelve a la posición de partida.

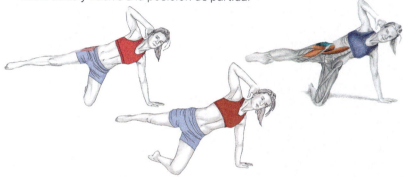

 Muscles Involved

Dynamic Muscles: The gluteus medius and tensor fasciae latae do the abduction of the leg. The pyramidalis and sartorius work to avoid the internal rotation that tends to occur as an effect of gravity and flexion of the hips. The iliopsoas, rectus anterior quadriceps and tensor fasciae latae intervene in flexing the hips (forward kick). Finally, the gluteus maximus and hamstrings allow the extension of the hips during the back kick.

Stabilizing Muscles: The abdominal transverse stabilizes the hips. The abdominal obliques support the midsection, and the trapezius keeps the shoulder girdle in place. The serrates, latissimus dorsi and pectoralis stabilize the upper trunk.

Others: All muscles, working together with other deeper muscles, keep the trunk and hips in the right position laterally. The anterior tibialis works while flexing the ankle, and the calf muscles while extending it.

Main Stretch: Lumbar Squareand hamstrings of the leg that kicks forward. Pectoralis and triceps of the raised arm with one hand behind your head.

Variations   1. On your Forearm

In this case you will need a box on which to support your forearm so as to keep your trunk at the right height. Since the base of support increases, this reduces intensity and provides a good stepping stone towards the basic exercise.

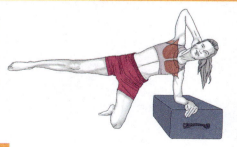

Adaptations

Do Variation 1 if you feel any wrist pain or instability.

You can place your hand on your forehead if the structure of your back makes it hard for you to keep it behind your head. This simple adaptation can greatly improve the position of the trunk.

Common Mistake: Twisting the Trunk

You must not allow the to droop downwards. To prevent this, imagine that you are trapped between two walls. This erroneous twist can place enormous strain on your lower back, and you should therefore shorten the path followed by your leg in the forward kick if you need to.

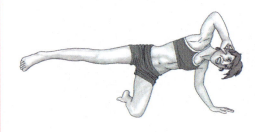

Common Mistake: Flexing the Hips

This failure of general stabilization results in destabilization of the hips. All the muscles must be active, each group doing its proper job.

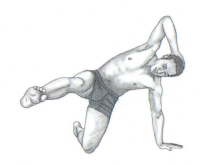

Notes: Let us again stress that the most important thing about the Pilates method is good form, however spectacular the result of the exercise may look. In this case, you must not sacrifice form for long leg movements, which depends on the flexibility of the muscles in the back of your neck, among numerous other factors.

2. Lying Down

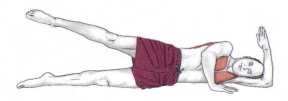

This way of doing the exercise turns it basically into Exercise 16 of Level 1, a side kick, although the placing of the hand behind your provides an interesting trunk stabilization component, especially as you perform the kicks.

1 Lower Body — One leg circles (6-1)

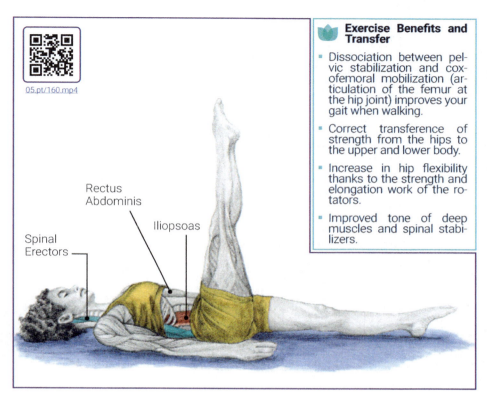

05.pt/160.mp4

Exercise Benefits and Transfer

- Dissociation between pelvic stabilization and coxofemoral mobilization (articulation of the femur at the hip joint) improves your gait when walking.
- Correct transference of strength from the hips to the upper and lower body.
- Increase in hip flexibility thanks to the strength and elongation work of the rotators.
- Improved tone of deep muscles and spinal stabilizers.

 Muscles Involved

Dynamic Muscles: In the leg doing the circles, the iliopsoas flexes the hips, which is the hardest part of the exercise. Therefore the strongest sensation of work is felt in the groin area. You will also feel a stretch in the iliopsoas of the leg that stays on the floor.

Stabilizing Muscles: The abdominal transverse keeps the hips still in a neutral position, which is a key aspect to avoid overloading the lower back. The neck muscles have to work hard to stabilize and elongate the neck without strain. The lower fibers of the trapezius are in charge of scapular stability.

Others: The obliques help "glue" the body to the floor. The glutes, quadriceps and calf muscles of the leg on the floor keep it outstretched and engaged.

Main Stretch: Gluteus maximus and hamstrings of the raised leg.

Variations 1. Knee of the Other Leg Flexed in the Air

The difficulty of the exercise can be increased by eliminating support from the leg that does not do the circles. The spinal stabilizers will be the muscles that work the hardest, as long as you are strict about form and do not move moving your head as you describe the leg circles.

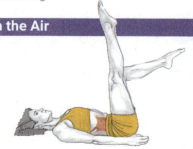

Keys to good form

- Stretch out your leg as if you wanted to touch the ceiling with your toes.
- Keep your trunk completely still, as if it were glued to the floor.
- Respect the natural curves of your back, always keeping your hips neutral.
- Do not make your circles too large, which can make your hips or trunk move.
- Avoid overloading your shoulders. All of the energy used in the upper back will be subtracted from the abdomen.
- Breathing: Inhale as you do half a circle and exhale as you finish that circle. You may also inhale during a full circle and exhale during the next.

How To?

1. Lie on your back, raise and stretch out one leg to the ceiling, keeping your ribcage closed and your core connected.

2. Do large or small leg circles from your hips, avoiding any movement of the spine.

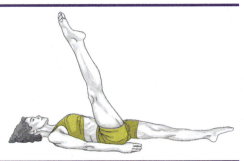

Adaptations

You can place a cushion under your hips to avoid lower back strain, (see Exercise 6 in Chapter 3 on Adapted Exercises).

 Notes: It is important to maintain coxofemoral articulation (union of the femur and flexible hip) to avoid negative motion patterns while walking, lighten the effect of arthrosis and avoid coaptations (locked joints) and other pelvic problems that can appear with time.

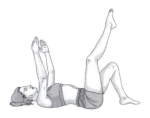

 Common Mistake: Loss of Spinal Elongation

Letting the lower back curve due to abdominal weakness. If this occurs, you need to feel the problem and correct your posture either by consciously reconnecting with the floor or by flexing the knee of the leg that is not describing circles and placing your foot on the floor.

2. Leg Inside a Ring

This results in more work for the iliopsoas and abdominal transverse, because doing the circles inside the ring, and therefore closer to the trunk, imposes a constraint. It will also stretch the lower fibers of the iliopsoas in the leg that is resting on the floor.

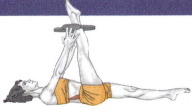

2 Lower Body — Heel squeeze prone (13-1)

Exercise Benefits and Transfer

- Increased strength in the glutes and hamstrings, parts of the body that constantly squashed while we sitting down, a frequent position during both work and leisure hours.
- Improved proprioception in prone positions.
- Dissociation between the work of the lower back and that of the hip extensors.

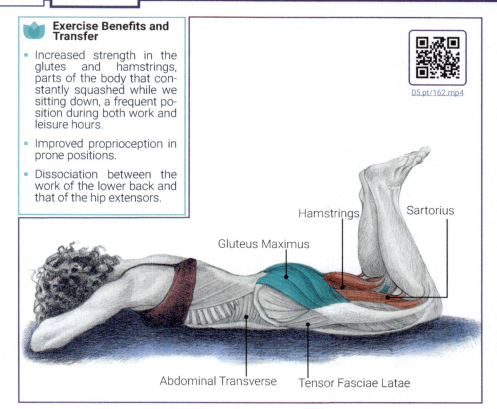

05.pt/162.mp4

 Muscles Involved

Dynamic Muscles: The femoral biceps (or hamstrings) produces external rotation of the knee. The deep fibers of the gluteus maximus, vastus medialis of the quadriceps and the major, middle and minor adductors do the work of adduction.

Stabilizing Muscles: The abdominal transverse is the main stabilizer of the hips and plays a key role in this exercise, since flexing the hips to generate more strength and aid the quadriceps is a common mistake. Cervical elongation is achieved thanks to the longus capitis and rectus anterior capitis.

Others: The abdominal obliques close the ribcage and the lower fibers of the trapezius stabilize the shoulder blades.

Main Stretch: Quadriceps.

 Notes: The variations increase or decrease the intensity of the exercises. In this case, Variation clearly intensifies the work because of the intermuscular coordination of both lower extremities. If this is under control, the ring will not move from its place, but it otherwise be very difficult to keep it between your ankles, even to the extent of preventing you from doing the exercise at all. If this happens, your should return to the original exercise until you feel both legs working with the same strength, the same rotation and the same angle of flexion in your knees.

Keys to good form

- Keep your neck elongated at the back and resist the temptation to raise your chin.
- Keep your shoulders, arms and pectorals relaxed.
- Do not separate your hips from the floor no matter what it takes to squeeze both heels together.
- Keep your trunk elongated, as if you wanted to touch the wall in front of you with the crown of your head.
- This should a slow and long squeeze. Don't be hasty.
- Breathing: inhale as you relax and exhale as you squeeze.

How To?

1. Lie face down with one hand on top of the other and your forehead on you're the backs of your hands. Flex and separate your knees and touch your heels together.

2. With your ribcage closed, core connected and hips touching the floor, squeeze both heels together as you flex your ankles (dorsal flexion).

3. Once you have squeezed your heels together, you can raise your knees of the floor, which increases the work done by the lower fibers of the glutes.

Adaptations

You can place a cushion under your hips if you have prominent abdomen, are a few months pregnant or suffer from lower back pain (see Exercise 2 in Chapter 3 on Adapted Exercises).

If your nose bothers or you find it hard to breathe with your face so close to the floor, you can put a cushion under your forehead to raise your head (see Exercise 22 in Chapter 3 on Adapted Exercises).

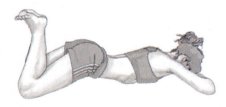

 Common Mistake: Flexing the Hips

This happens when you try to draw strength from your quadriceps and iliopsoas. The action involved in the exercise is difficult to control since the goal is only to squeeze. When you center on details and good form, however, you will begin to understand why flexing the hips reduces the benefits of this exercise.

Variations 1. With a ringbetween your ankles

This increases difficulty of the exercise due to the imbalance produced by the circular shape of the ring. This makes for an interesting variant once you have mastered the basic exercise.

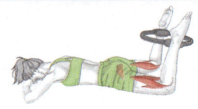

3 | Lower Body | One side leg kick (16-1)

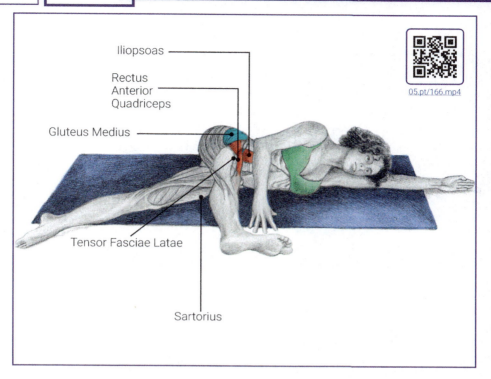

- Iliopsoas
- Rectus Anterior Quadriceps
- Gluteus Medius
- Tensor Fasciae Latae
- Sartorius

05.pt/166.mp4

Exercise Benefits and Transfer

- Development of the back muscles in a situation of minimum effort against gravity. Recommended for people with back conditions.
- Learning new motion patterns for the lateral lying position, which is common in the getting-up routine of seniors and of people with back conditions.
- Improved proprioception of the work done by the back muscles.

How To?

1. Start by lying on your side with one arm, trunk and legs completely outstretched and your head resting on the outstretched arm.
2. Raise your working leg as wide as your hips and kick forwards slowly, keeping your hips neutral and your spine elongated.
3. Return your leg to the starting position and kick backwards.

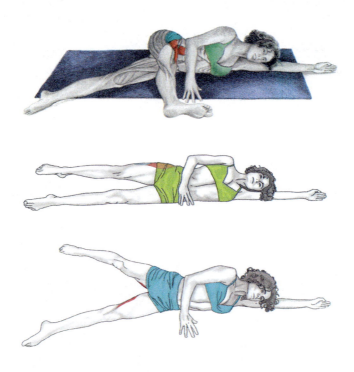

Variations 1. Hands behind your head

A much more intense and difficult variation that involves the back muscles especially. You should not do it unless you have mastered the principle of scapular stabilization.

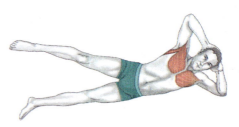

Keys to good form

- Imagine a line that goes from your pinky finger along your side and leg all the way down to your pinky toe. Support only this line on the floor, "gathering in" all the rest.
- As you kick, push your butt back (anteversion of the hips) to offset for any possible flexion.
- Stretch out your body and try to feel the stretch throughout the exercise, holding the tonic posture that will keep you lying steady on your side at all times.
- Breathing: Inhale in the starting position, exhale during the forwards kick, inhale as you return to starting position and exhale as you kick backwards.

Adaptations

Place a cushion between your arm and head if you feel shoulder pain (see Exercise 14 in Chapter 3 on Adapted Exercises).

Flex the leg of the supporting knee if you find yourself losing your balance (see Exercise 12 in Chapter 3 on Adapted Exercises).

 Notes: Exercises done lying on your side are generally very good for back conditions like scoliosis, because they stabilize the spine without causing stress. They also work as reinforcing therapy for lower back pain.

The term "kick" means a long, slow movement and not a brusque or sharp motion.

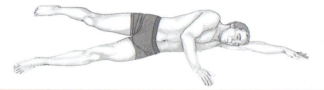

 Common Mistake: Poor Stabilization

This problem is caused by failure to engage the deep muscles of the trunk, which should accompany the vertebrae, the abdominal obliques, the latissimus dorsi, trapezius and pelvic stabilizers. The resulting feeling is that you are merely lying on the floor rather than supported by it as you should be.

 Muscles Involved

Dynamic Muscles: The gluteus maximus and tensor fasciae latae abduct the leg. The pyramidalis and sartorius work to control the tendency to rotate the leg internally, which results from the effect of gravity and flexing the hips. The iliopsoas, Gluteus Mediusand tensor fasciae latae are all involved in flexing the hips (forward kick). Finally, the gluteus maximus and hamstrings extend the hips in the back kick.

Stabilizing Muscles: The abdominal transverse stabilizes the hips, the abdominal obliques stabilize the midsection and the trapezius stabilizes the shoulder girdle.

Others: All of the muscles work together with other deep muscles to keep the trunk and hips in the right position. If you choose to flex your ankle during the forwards kick, you will be working on the anterior tibialis and stretching the calf muscles.

Main Stretch: QL and hamstring of the kicking leg.

4 Lower Body — Side leg series (17-1)

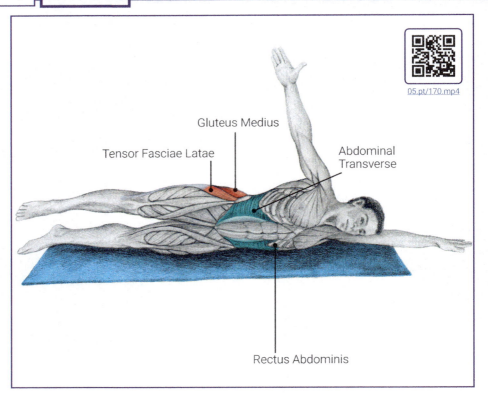

05.pt/170.mp4

Gluteus Medius
Tensor Fasciae Latae
Abdominal Transverse
Rectus Abdominis

 Exercise Benefits and Transfer

- Development of the back muscles in a situation of minimum effort against gravity. Recommended for people with back conditions.
- Learning new patterns of movement for the lateral lying position, which is common in the getting-up routine of seniors and people with back conditions.
- Increase in proprioception of the work performed by the muscles of your sides.
- Great workload for the abdominal obliques in an unusual position.

How To?

1. Lie on your side with one arm, your trunk and your legs completely outstretched and your head resting on your outstretched arm.

2. Raise your working leg about 10 cm wider than your hips.

3. Lower that leg until it touches the other one, always seeking elongation and muscular engagement.

4. Raise both legs while keeping them outstretched and lower them again to restart the exercise by raising only one leg.

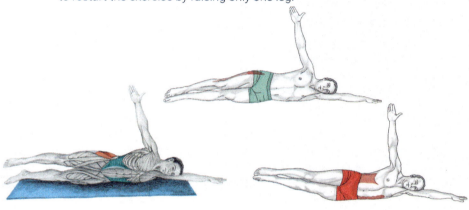

Adaptations

You can place a cushion between your arm and if you feel any shoulder pain (See Exercise 11 in Chapter 3 on Adapted Exercises).

 Notes: In all the exercises that involve moving your legs using your hips there is always the risk of the coxofemoral joint becoming locked. To prevent this and reap the maximum benefit from these exercises you must elongate your leg, as if you were trying to pull it out of its hip socket, stretching hard. This will work the muscles in eccentric contraction (stretching force/strength), avoiding strain and possible injury to the abductors and external rotators.

Variations 1. Pressing a Ring

Place a ring between your legs below the line of your ankle. It is very important to engage the muscle in the whole leg so as to prevent the adoption of a knock-kneed position. This variation includes work for the adductors.

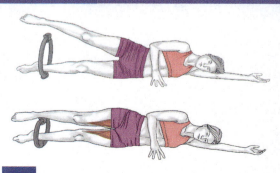

Keys to good form

- Imagine a line that goes from your pinky finger along your side and leg all the way down to your pinky toe. Support only this line on the floor, "gathering in" all the rest.
- Stretch out your body and try feel it this way throughout the exercise, without leaving the tonic posture that will keep you lying steady on your side.
- "Glue" your legs together, from groin to feet, as you raise both of them.
- The trunk should barely move, so the legs must be raised in a tightly constrained and controlled movement.
- Relax your shoulders to avoid straining your upper back.
- You need to elongate your neck from behind as you raise your legs. Cervical elongation helps resist the tendency to flex your spine.
- Breathing: Inhale in the neutral position, exhale as you raise one leg, inhale as you join both legs and exhale as you raise them together.

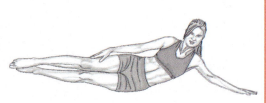

 Common Mistake: Flexing the Hips

This is caused by the feeling of weakness in the abdominal obliques, which usually makes people draw the strength from the quadriceps and iliopsoas, a gesture that necessarily causes flexion of the hips, largely cancelling out the benefits of the exercise.

 Muscles Involved

Dynamic Muscles: The gluteus medius and tensor fasciae latae abduct the leg. The gluteus medius, gluteus minor and tensor fasciae latae work to prevent the external rotation that is frequently made to draw strength from the quadriceps and iliopsoas. The minor oblique also works on the side of the raised leg and the major oblique on the opposite side. Finally, the anterior tibialis flexes the ankle.

Stabilizing Muscles: The abdominal transverse stabilizes the hips. The trapezius stabilizes the shoulder girdle. The spinal extensors prevent the trunk from flexing as the legs are raised. The gluteus maximus and hamstring keep the hips extended.

Others: The quadriceps of the supporting leg keeps the knee extended, while the gluteus maximus and hamstrings also extend the supporting hip on the floor.

Main Stretch: Adductors of the leg being raised (in Position 2). Tensor fasciae latae of the bottom leg in Position 3.

2. Expanding a Ring

Place both legs inside a ring, below the ankle line and try to expand or burst it. This variation works for the abductor muscles of the hips.

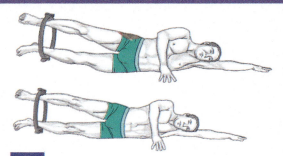

5 Lower Body — Single leg extension (20-1)

05.pt/172.mp4

Exercise Benefits and Transfer

- Strengthens and stretches the lower back muscles.
- Improved proprioception of abdominal work in a prone position.
- The variation is one of the most efficient exercises to work on the lower fibers of the gluteus maximus.

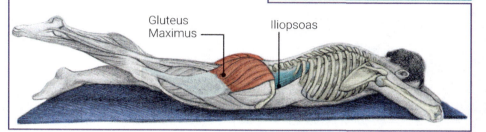

Gluteus Maximus — Iliopsoas

Keys to good form

- Kee the raised leg stretching backwards. This is not an elevation towards the ceiling.
- Imagine you were trying to pull your leg out of its hip socket.
- Keep your gaze fixed on the floor. This will keep your neck neutral and elongated.
- Avoid tensing your shoulders, neck and arms.
- Image that the elevation of your leg feeds off the power generated by your abs about 3 cm beneath your navel.
- Breathing: Inhale in the neutral position, exhale as you raise your leg, and inhale once more as you return to the neutral position.

How To?

1. Lie face down on the floor with your forehead resting on your hands and your elbows open and relaxed.
2. Raise one leg, extending it and activating all the muscles from hip to toe.
3. Lower the leg without losing the muscular engagement you have achieved. Do not relax as you return your leg to the floor but maintain the working position.

Variations 1. Flexing and Raising the Knees

Separate your legs a little more, flex your knees and raise them a little from the ground, as if to touch your glutes with your heels. This variation will work your gluteus maximus and hamstrings more intensely.

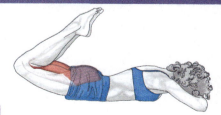

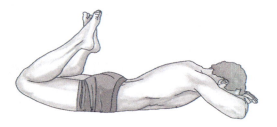

 Common Mistake: Drawing power from your back

If you seek to draw power from your back you will impede spinal elongation, shortening the muscle chains and eliminating the benefits from the exercise. You will also sacrifice stability in your shoulder girdle and strain muscle groups that have nothing to do with hip extension.

Adaptations

Place a cushion under your hips to avoid flexing them and straining your lower back (see Exercise 2 in Chapter 3 on Adapted Exercises).

Place a cushion under your forehead if you find the prone position makes breathing uncomfortable (see Exercise 22 in Chapter 3 on Adapted Exercises).

 Muscles Involved

Dynamic Muscles: The muscles of the lower back, gluteus maximus and hamstrings extend the hips as you raise your legs. The calf muscles work perform the plantar flexion or extension of the ankle.

Stabilizing Muscles: The abdominal transverse, longissimus dorsi, quadriceps and spinal transverses stabilize the trunk and hips, and help elongate the upper body. The lower fibers of the trapezius act as scapular stabilizers.

Others: The posterior deltoid keeps the elbows separated, and the neck muscles, longus capitis and rectus anterior capitis, elongate the cervical spine.

Main Stretch: Iliopsoas.

 Notes: Elongating the trunk and the legs is key to avoiding lower back strain. Imagine the process: the muscles of your upper body pull forwards and those of your lower body pull backwards, leaving the lower back in the middle, so that both its upper and lower fibers stretch.

6 Lower Body — Prone gluteo (27-1)

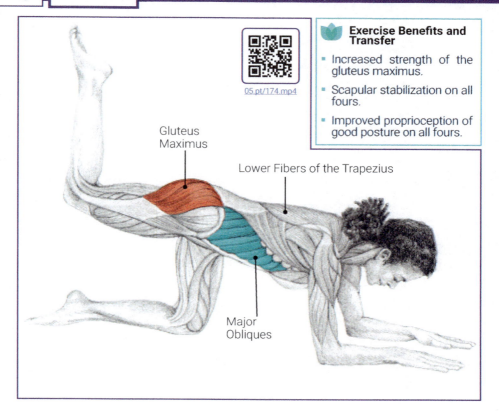

Exercise Benefits and Transfer
- Increased strength of the gluteus maximus.
- Scapular stabilization on all fours.
- Improved proprioception of good posture on all fours.

 Muscles Involved

Dynamic Muscles: Mainly the glutes; to a lesser degree, the hamstrings.

Stabilizing Muscles: The abdominal transverse keeps the hips neutral and the obliques intervene in stabilizing the trunk. The lower fibers of the trapezius guarantee scapular stabilization.

Others: The serrates add in the right location of the upper back.

Main Stretch: Quadriceps and iliopsoas.

Variations 1. With Outstretched Leg

Raise one leg, with the knee extended, to the height of your trunk. From there, raise and lower it just like in the original exercise.

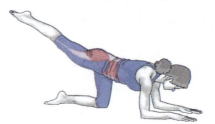

Keys to good form

- Keep your lower abdomen (abdominal transverse muscle) active throughout the exercise.
- Try not to look forwards or backwards in order to attain complete axial elongation.
- The energy for moving the leg should come from your glutes, not from your back.
- Keep your lower back and hips still throughout the exercise.
- The movement of the leg is minimal, but the activation of the glute is maximal.
- Breathing: Exhale during descent, inhale during ascent.

Notes: You should do a good workout for your glutes every day. The exercises concerned should not involve articulation of the lower back but should increase the strength of your glutes, which are key to the movement.

How To?

1. Begin on all fours with forearms flat on the floor, your spine neutral and one leg raised with the knee flexed 90 degrees.
2. Keep your knee flexed as you raise and lower your leg.

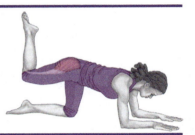

Adaptations

If you have problems supporting your knees on the floor, you could do this exercise standing up (see Exercise 16 in Pilates Standing Exercises).

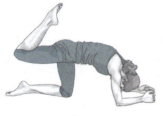

 Common Mistake: Dorsal Hyperkyphosis

Excessive roundness of the upper back and scapular destabilization. This habit causes strain and potentially injuries to the upper back, neck and shoulders.

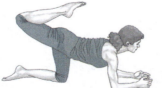

 Common Mistake: Lumbar Hyperlordosis

Excessive arching of the lower back and opening of the ribcage. This happens when you stop thinking about your abdomen and pay all your attention to your glutes.

2. Heel to Glute

In approaching your glute with your heel you stretch out your quadriceps more and work the lower fibers of your gluteus maximus and your hamstrings harder. Be aware of spinal neutrality, since this is the most intense variation.

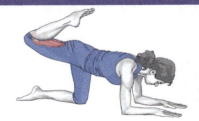

7   Lower Body   The bridge (2-2)

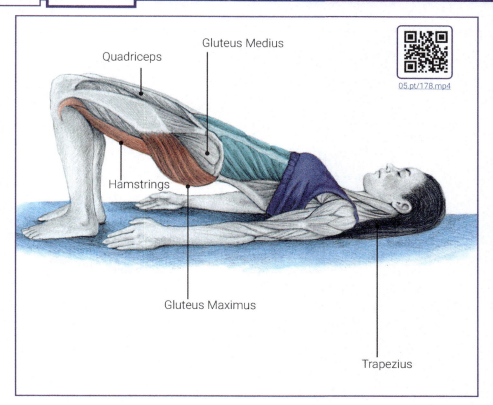

 Exercise Benefits and Transfer

- Strengthens the posterior chain.
- Learning the concept of neutral hips and pelvic stabilization in a supine raised position.
- As long as spinal articulation is correct, this exercise will help destress a painful lower back.
- Relaxation.
- Teaches dynamic elongation of the spine.

Keys to good form

- Keep your gaze on the ceiling right above your eyes.
- Keep your neck elongated, as a prolongation of your spine, feeling its extension from behind as if someone were pulling at the back of your skull.
- The four steps of articulation ensure order in the raising and lowering of the trunk, but this can also be done in a fluid and continuous way.
- Keep your heels close to your hips, but not excessively. This will help you to articulate better.
- Imagine that someone is about to sit on your abdomen, which must be prepared to support that weight.
- Breathing: Inhale in the starting position, exhale as you raise your trunk, and inhale as you lower it.

How To?

1. Lie on your back with flexed knees, your feet pinned to the floor and arms by your sides.
2. Raise your trunk into the air following a four-stage pattern. First the hips are passed from neutral to raised by retroversion, then the lower back is raised, then a small part of the upper back, then the rest of the upper back.
3. Lower your trunk following the same four-step pattern in reverse order.

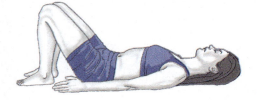 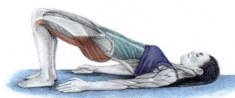

Variations 1. Feet on a Cylinder

The exercise is done exactly in the same manner, but you have to keep the cylinder from moving. Since this is an unstable support (it is round and will roll), the workload of the posterior muscles, especially the glutes and hamstrings, is greatly intensified.

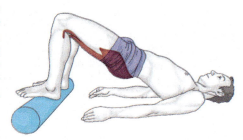

Adaptations

To avoid elevation beyond what is adequate, place your feet on an elevated support. This variation removes the sensation that the bridge is not rising enough and moderates elevation of the trunk and opening of the ribcage (see Exercise 16 in Chapter 3 on Adapted Exercises).

You can place an arc beneath your lower back and hips to do Variation 1 if your are suffering from lower back pain (see Exercise 17 in Chapter 3 on Adapted Exercises).

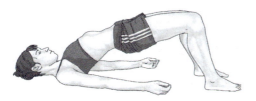

 Common Mistake: Lumbar Hyperlordosis and Open Ribcage

This happens when the pattern of articulation throughout the rise is not right or disorderly, and if you try to drive the movement only using your back muscles but not your abs.

Notes: A well-executed bridge should describe an ascending straight line from shoulders to knees. Once the movement is completed, the effort should be felt only in the glutes and hamstrings. The quadriceps can also be felt, but only on a secondary level.

Avoid separating your knees, which should remain hip-width apart, as should the whole of your legs. If you open your legs too wide, you will cancel out most of the work done by the lower fibers of the gluteus maximus.

 Muscles Involved

Dynamic Muscles: The paravertebrals articulate the spine during both ascent and descent. The pyramidalis, crural square, hamstrings and gluteus maximus do the initial retroversion of the hips. The rectus abdominis flexes the spine as the trunk descends.

Stabilizing Muscles: The lower fibers of the trapezius stabilize the shoulder blades so that the shoulders do not approach the ears. The abdominal obliques close the ribcage.

Others: The quadriceps should lengthen, and be felt to lengthen to aid the other muscle groups in keeping the hips neutral in the air at the end of the exercise.

Main Stretch: Iliopsoas.

2. Bridge with Kick

Raise the bridge and keep it in place. Stretch one leg forwards, diagonally, then raise it to your trunk as you flex your ankle.

Lower your leg, without approaching the floor too much, while stretching out your ankle. This variation works for the quadriceps and iliopsoas of the active leg, as well as for all the muscles mentioned above.

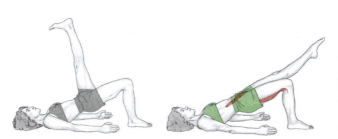

8 Lower Body — One leg kick (4-2)

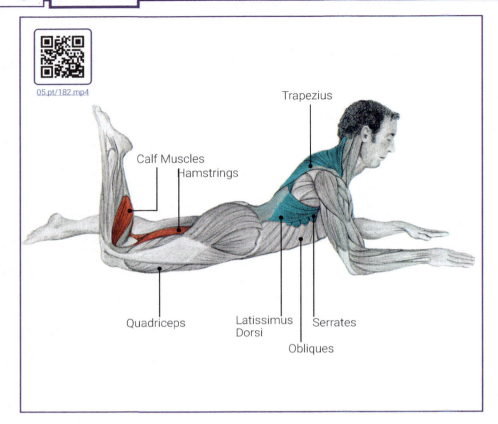

05.pt/182.mp4

Labels: Trapezius, Calf Muscles, Hamstrings, Quadriceps, Latissimus Dorsi, Obliques, Serrates

Exercise Benefits and Transfer

- Strengthens the outstretched lower back.
- Improves proprioception of the obliques and abdominal transverse in prone position.
- This exercise will help you understand scapular stabilization with forearm support in a prone position, which is common during active rest.

How To?

1. Lie face down supporting yourself on your forearms with your trunk and legs fully elongated.
2. Flex one knee to 90 degrees, keeping your ankle extended.
3. Open up the flexion angle and flex 90 degrees once more, this time with the ankle flexed.
4. Stretch out your knee without disengaging the muscles and do the same exercise with the other leg.

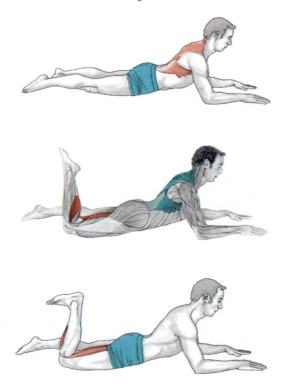

Variations 1. Support on your hands

In this variation it is not the forearms that are supported on the floor, but the hands. The triceps play a key role.

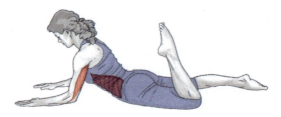

Keys to good form

- Flex your knee as if there were resistance to overcome.
- Try to free your leg from your hip, pulling back as you flex your knee.
- Keep your gaze diagonal towards the floor maintain a neutral, elongated neck.
- Every muscle in your trunk should work to achieve maximum elongation and stabilization.
- Breathing: Inhale in the neutral position. Exhale twice, once during the knee flexion with extended ankle and once more during the second knee flexion with flexed ankle. Inhale as you return to the neutral position.

Adaptations

Place a cushion beneath your hips to avoid flexing them and straining your lower back (see Exercise 2 in Chapter 3 on Adapted Exercises).

Place a cushion under your forehead if you find breathing uncomfortable in the prone position (see Exercise 22 in Chapter 3 on Adapted Exercises).

You can place a cushion under your thighs just below your knees to protect your kneecaps (see Exercise 19 in Chapter 3 on Adapted Exercises).

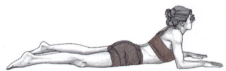

 Common Mistake:

Failure to concentrate on the stabilization work done by the upper body can lead to ignoring the position of your shoulder blades with the result that your shoulders approach your ears, reducing the discal space of the cervical spine. This will quickly overload trapezius, forcing you to give up the exercise.

 Notes: Scapular Destabilization.

Imagine that you have to press a foam cushion with your foot during the kick with flexed ankle. This foam offers considerable resistance which you must overcome with the strength of your hamstrings. However, your foot must not reach your glute, but is restrained before that. This is the intention with which you need to approach this apparently simple but exercise, which is actually quite complex in practice. If you cannot generate this strength with braking, you will barely feel the work of the hamstrings.

 Muscles Involved

Dynamic Muscles: The hamstrings flex the knees and the calf muscles and the anterior tibialis flexes and extends the ankles. The quadriceps extends the knees after the kicks.

Stabilizing Muscles: The serrates, rhomboids, latissimus dorsi, trapezius and spinal erectors keep the trunk elongated and shoulder blades stabilized. The abdominal transverse and obliques reduce any strain in the middle and lower back.

Others: The longus capitis and rectus anterior capitis elongate the cervical spine. The triceps assist in stabilizing the shoulders and elbows.

Main Stretch: Quadriceps and iliopsoas.

9 Lower Body — Hinge (15-2)

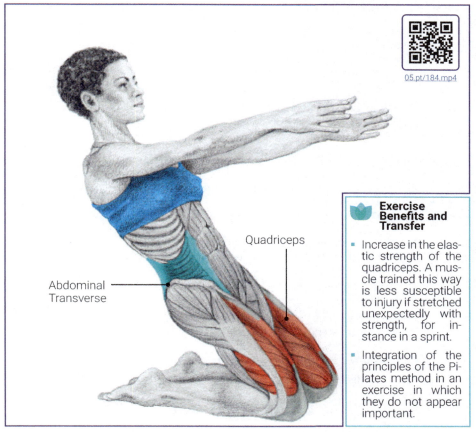

05.pt/184.mp4

Quadriceps

Abdominal Transverse

Exercise Benefits and Transfer

- Increase in the elastic strength of the quadriceps. A muscle trained this way is less susceptible to injury if stretched unexpectedly with strength, for instance in a sprint.
- Integration of the principles of the Pilates method in an exercise in which they do not appear important.

 Muscles Involved

Dynamic Muscles: The stars of this exercise are the quadriceps, which are responsible for extending the knees.

Stabilizing Muscles: The abdominal transverse and abdominal obliques are the muscles that keep the trunk stable in the front, while the QL does so at the back.

Others: The glutes may be activated during the rise to avoid anteversion of the hips, but this should not be the main focus of attention because that would make the hips pass to retroversion and lose their neutral position.

Main Stretch: Quadriceps.

Variations 1. With Outstretched Arm

Raise an arm as you lean your trunk and legs backwards. This arm must not surpass the head line. By increasing the lever of the trunk, you will make the exercise harder for the legs. You will also active the abdominal obliques on the side of the raised arm.

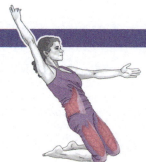

Keys to good form

- Keep your whole body like a steel plate, especially while you move.
- Keep your eyes front.
- Avoid brusque movements.
- Keep the range of movement within your ability. It is better to descend a little and in a controlled fashion than to abandon the principles of the method on the way.
- Breathing: Since this exercise is hard in both its stages, you can have your pick. Conventionally, you should inhale during descent and exhale during ascent.

 Common Mistake: Extending the Hips

Allowing your hips to come forwards like a matador will strain your lower back and detract from the work done by the quadriceps.

How To?

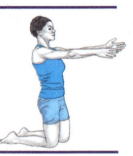

1. Start from a kneeling position stretching the crown of your head up towards the ceiling and apply all the principles of the Pilates method.
2. Increase the flexion of your knees, leaning your trunk backwards with your arms extended forwards.
3. Return to the starting position. You can keep your arms extended after starting the exercise.

Adaptations

If kneeling on the floor hurts, you can place a cushion beneath your knees.

If feel any discomfort in your feet, you can place a rolled-up futon or blanket under them (see Exercise 15 in Chapter 3 on Adapted Exercises).

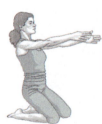

 Common Mistake: Flexing the Hips

This increases enormously the flexion of the knees and can cause injury because of the very tight angle at which you will be working.

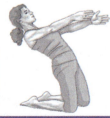

 Common Mistake: Extending the Hips

Allowing your hips to come forwards like a matador will strain your lower back and detract from the work done by the quadriceps.

2. Oblique

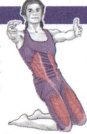

Twist your trunk, accompanied by your arms, while keeping your hips facing forwards. This increases the workload for the abdominal obliques without flexing the trunk.

10 Lower Body — Rocking (8-3)

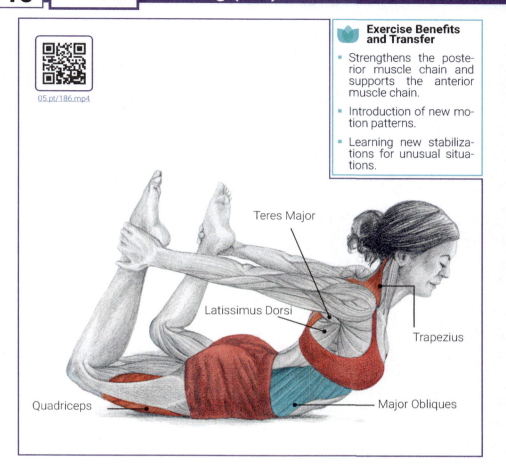

05.pt/186.mp4

Exercise Benefits and Transfer

- Strengthens the posterior muscle chain and supports the anterior muscle chain.
- Introduction of new motion patterns.
- Learning new stabilizations for unusual situations.

Labels: Teres Major, Latissimus Dorsi, Trapezius, Quadriceps, Major Obliques

 Notes: Breathing is key in this exercise. As you exhale, notice how you obtain more support and power to help you raise your trunk. You will need to do a few repetitions to find the right balance of weight between your upper and lower body. This is key to finding good support for your hips

 Common Mistake: Failure to extend your knees

This will keep you from rising and surely force you to draw strength from your lower back.

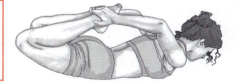

Keys to good form

- Keep your quadriceps steadily engaged while trying to extend your knees. This is key to raising your trunk.
- In the rocking option, think of yourself as a seesaw with your legs and the front of your body as the rocker.
- Keep your eyes front in the raised position to avoid straining your neck.
- Breathing: Inhale in the starting position, and exhale while extending your knees and raising your trunk.

How To?

1. Lying face down, flex your knees and grasp your ankles and the front of your feet.

2. Without relaxing your grip, try to extend your knees. You will be unable to do so, of course, but this action will result in an enormous extension of your spine, thereby raising your trunk.

3. Optionally, rock back and forth, keeping a steady momentum.

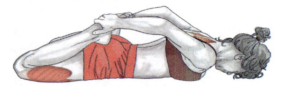

Adaptations

You may try first a Swan Dive (Exercise 3 of Level 3) or, if you want to do a complete progression, a dorsal extension (Exercise 2 of Level 1).

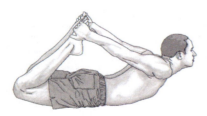

 Common Mistake: Raising the chin

This happens when you cannot find the strength to raise your trunk. In this case, you should first study the exercise technique and then try to draw power from your quadriceps as you extend your knees.

 Muscles Involved

Dynamic Muscles: Minimally the quadriceps in the small movement involved in the "intention" to extend the knees.

Stabilizing Muscles: The rhomboids, trapezius and spinal erectors keep the trunk elongated and the shoulder blades stabilized. The connection of the abdominal transverse muscle protects the lower back. The lumbar muscles and glutes keep the body boat-shaped.

Others: The longus capitis and rectus anterior capitis elongate the cervical spine.

Main Stretch: Anterior muscle chain and antepulsors of the shoulders.

1 Upper Body — Breast Stroke (2-1)

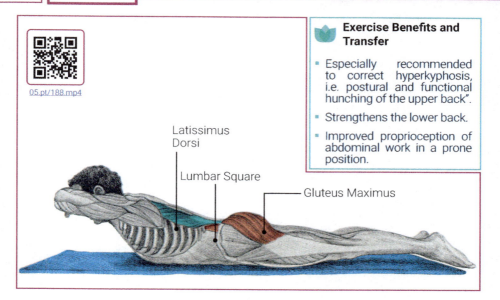

05.pt/188.mp4

Exercise Benefits and Transfer

- Especially recommended to correct hyperkyphosis, i.e. postural and functional hunching of the upper back".
- Strengthens the lower back.
- Improved proprioception of abdominal work in a prone position.

Labels: Latissimus Dorsi, Lumbar Square, Gluteus Maximus

Keys to good form

- More than rising, you have to grow forwards and up.
- Keep your on the floor throughout so that your neck stays neutral and elongated.
- Shoulders, neck and arms must remain free from tension.
- Image that the power to raise your trunk comes from your abdomen.
- Breathing: Inhale in position 1 and exhale in position 2.

 Notes: The most important thing to seek in this exercise is elongation of the trunk, rather raising it straight up. The legs must be literally "glued" to the floor to avoid activating the lower back to far, which you should work rather in the elongation phase.

 Muscles Involved

Dynamic Muscles: The quadratus lumborum increases the curve of the lower back and the longissimus dorsi elongates the spine. The spinal transverse muscles extend the spine. The rectus abdominis works in eccentric contraction, supporting the elevation.

Stabilizing Muscles: The glutes, hamstrings and abdominal transverse stabilize the hips and aid in attaining a "long" lower body. The lower fibers of the trapezius stabilize the shoulder blades.

Others: The posterior deltoids keep the elbows separated.

Main Stretch: Rectus abdominis.

How To?

1. Lie face down (on your chest) with forehead on your hands and your elbows open and relaxed.

2. Extend your spine, trying to grow forwards at the same time. Keep your spine elongated as you lower your trunk. Your hands should be the last body part to touch the floor.

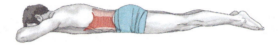

Adaptations

You can place a cushion under your hips to avoid flexing them, which would result in lower back overload (see Exercise 2 in Chapter 3 on Adapted Exercises).

You can squeeze a ball between your thighs if you find your legs open excessively (see Exercise 18 in Chapter 3 on Adapted Exercises).

Place a cushion under your forehead if you find breathing uncomfortable in the prone position (see Exercise 22 in Chapter 3 on Adapted Exercises).

 Common Mistake: Chin up and shoulders close to ears

Translated into the principles of the Pilates method, these two gestures are caused by poor cervical elongation and scapular stabilization. They cause overload in the upper back and neck, voiding the exercise of most of its benefits.

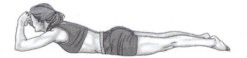

Variations 1. With Breast Stroke After Rising

This lengthens the time for which the trunk is kept raised, which in turn increases the intensity of the exercise. It is especially recommended in minor cases of scoliosis (spinal curvature) and for dorsal kyphosis (hunched back). Pull your arms backwards as if swimming the breaststroke, seeking maximum elongation in their final path, as if you were trying to touch the back wall with your fingers.

This works all of the medial back muscles.

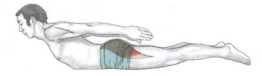

1 Relax — Shell stretch (22-1)

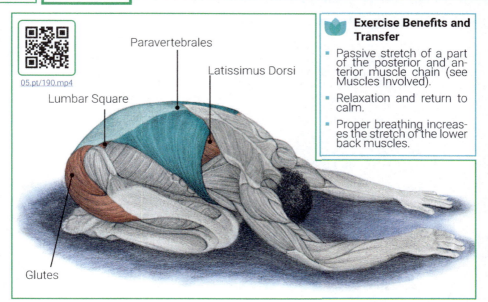

Exercise Benefits and Transfer

- Passive stretch of a part of the posterior and anterior muscle chain (see Muscles Involved).
- Relaxation and return to calm.
- Proper breathing increases the stretch of the lower back muscles.

Labels: Paravertebrales, Latissimus Dorsi, Lumbar Square, Glutes

05.pt/190.mp4

 Muscles Involved

Dynamic Muscles: This exercise does not involve any dynamic or stabilizing muscles, because the purpose is relaxation. Therefore, you should let your body react naturally, respecting its biomechanical patterns.

Main Stretch: The quadratus lumborum, gluteus maximus and flexors of the neck stretch passively. The latissimus dorsi stretches as well if you choose the option with outstretched arms. Finally, if ankle structure allows it, the dorsal flexors will stretch as well.

 Notes: In some schools in Spain, this exercise is known as "bolita" (little ball), in others as shell stretch or "concha" (seashell). Over time, the author of the original Spanish book has found that the term "bolita" is more easily understood by Spaniards and that it can be applied to the sitting position, lying on one's side or lying supine while holding the legs from behind.

Variations   1. Arms behind   2. Sitting down

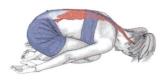   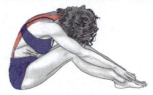

Place your arms behind your thighs, staying completely relaxed. You can also gather them by flexing your elbows and putting your hands on the hollow between your chest and neck. In these variations you no longer stretch your latissimus dorsi but they avoid shoulder pain.

Sit and flex your trunk, keeping neck, arms and shoulders relaxed. The breathing pattern is the same. The only difference is that you do not stretch either stretch your latissimus dorsi or the dorsal flexors of your ankles.

Keys to good form

- Support the front of your skull (not your forehead) on the floor. This will keep your neck extended.
- If the position is uncomfortable or painful for your knees, ankles or toes, look at the adapted exercises that address these issues. The shell stretch is an exercise that you should keep up over time, seeking to improve your comfort level.
- If your shoulders hurt in the basic position, look for a painless variation.
- If abdominal volume hinders the shell stretch position, look for a variation.
- Breathing: Breathing should be relaxed and gentle, sending air to the lower and posterior parts of the back. Both as you inhale and exhale, imagine locks opening in your lower back, letting water flow through a channel.

How To?

1. Sit down with your glutes planted on your heels and your knees on the floor. Flex your trunk forward with your arms out and your head resting on the floor.

Adaptations

If your knees hurt, you can place a rolled-up mat or towel in the hollow behind them (see Exercise 14 in Chapter 3 on Adapted Exercises).

If you cannot do a prone shell stretch because of abdominal volume, choose Variation 2, which is done sitting down.

If your ankles or toes hurt, you can place a rolled-up mat or towel beneath your feet or ankles (see Exercise 15 in Chapter 3 on Adapted Exercises).

If your shoulders hurt because of the forward-facing outstretched arms, you can gather your arms in between your chest and neck, or move them backwards (see Variation 1).

 Common Mistake: Wrong Placement of Head and Ankles

You need to be careful only with the placement of your head, which should be supported on the front of your skull just ahead of the crown and not on your forehead. Keep your ankles aligned or facing inwards if you feel any pain. They must not be placed so as to face outward, which could hurt lateral internal ligament of the knees.

3. Widely separated knees

If you have a prominent abdomen or are pregnant, you can keep doing the shell stretch for as long as the position with separated knees feels comfortable (this is like doing a "frog" stance). There are no pregnancy issues here, because the position increases the flexibility of the hips. This may not be possible when the reason for doing this variation is abdominal volume due to overweight.

4. Supine

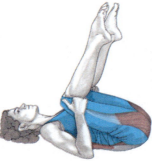

Hug your legs with your knees flexed and relax your whole body.

Stretches/Relaxation

Quadriceps (1)

How To?

Lying on your front, with hips glued to the floor.
Flex your knees and, with help from the hand on either side, pull your heels to your glutes.

Hamstrings and Calf Muscles

How To?

Lying on your back with the supporting leg flexed.
You can maintain a minimal knee flexion to stretch your hamstrings, but you will have to extend it and flex your ankle to stretch your calf muscles.

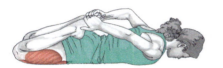

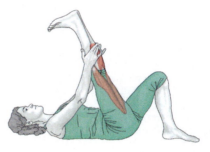

Gluteus Maximus and Quadratus Lumborum (3)

How To?

Lie on your back.
Flex your knees and grasp them from behind to pull them towards your chest.

Gluteus Medius and Sides (4)

How To?

Lie on your back with your palms up.
Bring your knees towards your chest and twist your trunk until your legs rest on the floor.

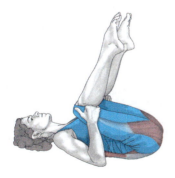

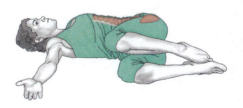

Stretches/Relaxation

Dorsal (5)

How To?

Sit down.
Flex your knees and hug your legs letting your head drop without tension or tension in your neck.

Pectoral (6)

How To?

Sitting cross-legged, in the lotus position or on a chair if you prefer.
Raise your arm with the elbow flexed and palm facing forwards.
Pull your arm backwards, keeping your elbow and shoulder at the same height, while you pull the fibers of your pectoral muscle towards the sternum in the opposite direction to your elbow.

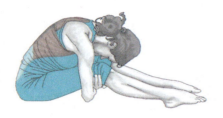
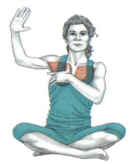

Anterior Chain (7)

How To?

Prepare a rolled-up blanket, a foam ball or a medium cushion.
Lie down facing the ceiling your knees flexed and feet planted on the floor. Raise your trunk as if you were doing Exercise 2 of Level 2, the Bridge, placing the blanket (or other support) under your hips.
Undo the bridge while letting all your body weight rest between the floor and the blanket.

Posterior Chain (8)

How To?

Lie face down on the floor on a rounded object (arc, rolled-up blanket, etc.) place under your hips and abdomen.
Let all your body weight rest.

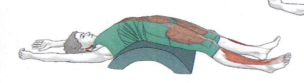

Stretches/Relaxation

Lateral Chain (9)

How To?

Lie down on one side on an arc or rolled-up blanket or mat placed under your hips and side.
Stretch out your arms on either side of your head and let all your body weight rest.

Shoulders and Trapezius (10)

How To?

Sitting down with legs crossed, entwine your fingers behind your back.
Pull your hands downwards and backwards, feeling your shoulders and thorax open at the front.

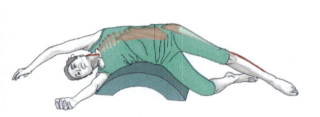
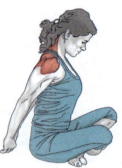

Stretches/Relaxation

Neck (11)

Stretch for the back of the neck

How To?

Maintaining axial elongation (i.e. trying to touch the ceiling with the crown of your head), flex your neck forwards as if you were trying to touch your throat with your chin.

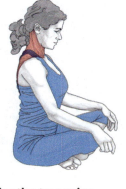

Stretch for the sides of the neck

How To?

Maintaining axial elongation, flex your neck sideways, bringing your ear to your shoulder.

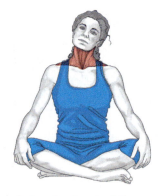

Stretch for the trapezius

How To?

Maintaining axial elongation, twist your neck, then flex it while bringing your lower jaw down towards your throat.

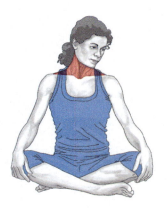

Stretch for the front of the neck

How To?

Maintaining axial elongation, raise your chin while stretching the back of your neck as far as you can. This should produce a feeling of elongation from behind and stretching of the skin from in front.

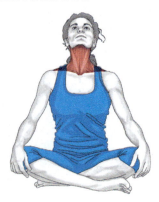

1 Standing Pilates — Ab prep (1-1)

How To?

1. From a kneeling position, with your hands behind your neck, flex your trunk without losing axial elongation.
2. Return to the starting position by extending your trunk until you have brought your spine back to the neutral position.

Muscles Involved

- Rectus abdominis.
- Abdominal transverse.
- Gluteus maximus
- Hamstrings

Main Stretch

Quadratus Lumborum.

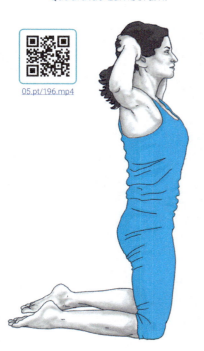

05.pt/196.mp4

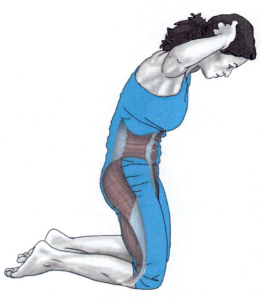

Breathing

Inhale in the starting position, exhale as you flex your trunk and inhale as you return to the starting position.

Differences and Similarities with the Floor Exercise

It will be difficult to do full abdominal work because of the need to keep your hips neutral. However, keeping your hips neutral will involve your glutes and hamstrings.

2 Standing Pilates — Breast stroke (2-1)

How To?

1. From a standing position, with your hands behind your head and your knees slightly flexed to avoid locking.
2. Extend your spine, keeping your ribcage closed and your eyes front, then return to the elongated starting position.

Muscles Involved
- Medial dorsals
- Rectus abdominis
- Oblique abdominals

Main Stretch

Rectus abdominis

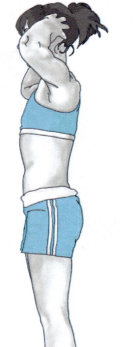
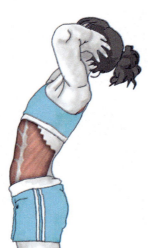

05.pt/197.mp4

Breathing

nhale in the starting position, exhale during spinal extension and inhale as you return to starting position.

Differences and Similarities with the Floor Exercise

Since there is no pressure from the floor on the front of the body, the standing position makes it easier to extend the spine. However, this easier execution can produce negative results if you fail to maintain good pelvic stabilization.

Half roll back (4-1)

Standing Pilates — 3

How To?

1. Start from a standing position with your arms raised.
2. Flex your trunk and push your hips back, then return to the neutral elongated position.

05.pt/198.mp4

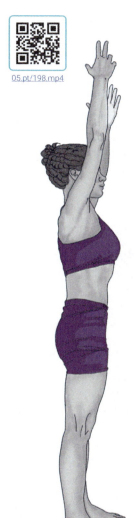

Main Stretch

Quadratus Lumborum.

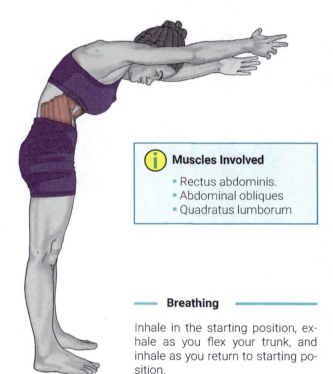

Muscles Involved

- Rectus abdominis.
- Abdominal obliques
- Quadratus lumborum

Breathing

Inhale in the starting position, exhale as you flex your trunk, and inhale as you return to starting position.

Differences and Similarities with the Floor Exercise

It may seem confusing that the movement is done forwards, instead of backwards as in the floor exercise. The mechanics of the standing exercise mean that the rectus abdominis works in concentric contraction during the half roll back and eccentric contraction when return to the starting position, which is the opposite pattern to the floor exercise.

4 Standing Pilates — Roll up (5-1)

How To?

1. Start from a standing position with your arms by your sides.
2. Flex your trunk deeply and bring your hips back, placing your arms parallel to the floor behind your, then return to the elongated starting position.

Muscles Involved
- Rectus abdominis
- Quadratus lumborum

Main Stretch

Spinal erectors, QL, anterior deltoids, hamstrings and gluteus maximus.

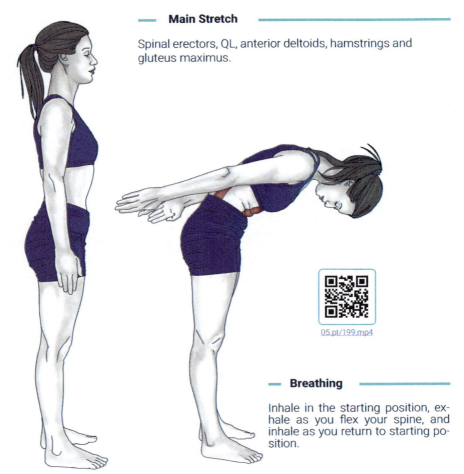

05.pt/199.mp4

Breathing

Inhale in the starting position, exhale as you flex your spine, and inhale as you return to starting position.

Differences and Similarities with the Floor Exercise

The trunk is flexed forwards from the standing position, so that the rectus abdominis works in concentric contraction in the half roll back and in eccentric contraction as your return to the starting position.

5 Standing Pilates — One-leg circles (6-1)

How To?

1. Start from a standing position with arms outstretched forwards and one leg extended and raised.
2. Do circles with your raised leg, clockwise and counterclockwise.

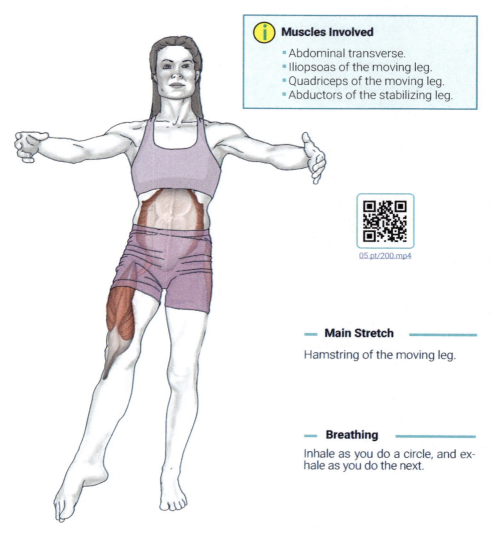

Muscles Involved

- Abdominal transverse.
- Iliopsoas of the moving leg.
- Quadriceps of the moving leg.
- Abductors of the stabilizing leg.

05.pt/200.mp4

Main Stretch

Hamstring of the moving leg.

Breathing

Inhale as you do a circle, and exhale as you do the next.

Differences and Similarities with the Floor Exercise

The work of the rectus abdominis is not so evident, and you will notice that of the abdominal transverse and iliopsoas much more. There is also work for the quadriceps of the moving leg and the abductors of the stabilizing leg as you balance.

6 Standing Pilates — Twist (7-1)

How To?

1. Start from a standing position with legs apart and arms outstretched in a cross.
2. Rotate your trunk accompanying the movement with your arms and gaze. Your hips must stay still, facing forwards throughout.
3. Return to the elongated starting position.

> **Muscles Involved**
> - Minor oblique on the side of the Twist.
> - Major oblique on the side opposite the Twist.

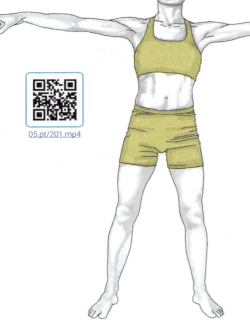

05.pt/201.mp4

Main Stretch

Spinal erectors, quadratus lumborum, anterior deltoids, hamstrings and gluteus maximus.

Breathing

Inhale in the starting position, exhale as you Twist your trunk, inhale as you return to starting position.

Differences and Similarities with the Floor Exercise

The difficulty of keeping the trunk elongated while sitting down is eliminated, but you will have concentrate more on keeping your hips and legs still.

7 Standing Pilates — Rolling like a ball (8-1)

How To?

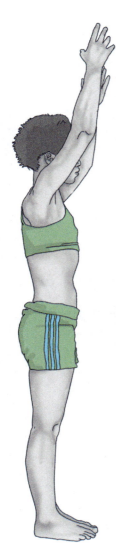

1. Start from a standing position with your arms raised.
2. Flex your trunk, hips and one knee until you can grasp your ankle between your hands.
3. Return to the starting position, undoing the ball progressively as you go.

Main Stretch

Spinal erectors.

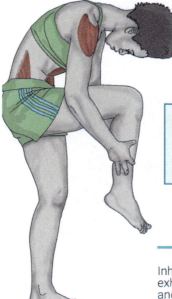

05.pt/202.mp4

Muscles Involved

- Rectus abdominis
- Iliopsoas
- Deltoid

Breathing

Inhale in the starting position, exhale as you flex your trunk, and inhale as you return to the starting position.

Differences and Similarities with the Floor Exercise

The main differences lie in the dynamic movement of the arms, the absence of contact with the floor against your back and the need to maintain balance. This is a more complex and intense exercise than the traditional Rolling Like a Ball. However, it still offers the benefit of stretching the spinal erectors.

8 Standing Pilates

One leg stretch (9-1)

How To?

1. From a standing position, with one leg raised and flexed and hands touching either side of your knee.
2. Stretch the flexed leg forwards and raise your arms.

Muscles Involved

- Abdominal transverse
- Iliopsoas of the dynamic leg
- Quadriceps of the dynamic leg
- Glutes of the stabilizing leg
- Spinal erectors

Main Stretch

Posterior chain on the side of the raised leg.

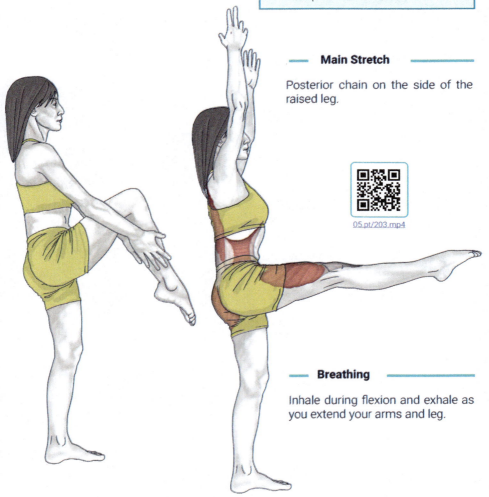

05.pt/203.mp4

Breathing

Inhale during flexion and exhale as you extend your arms and leg.

Differences and Similarities with the Floor Exercise

This exercise is completely different when it comes to the work of the rectus abdominis, which in this case stabilizes the trunk. This exercise implies a considerable stretch of the posterior chain on the side of the outstretched leg, and it simultaneously strengthens the anterior chain on the same side.

9 Standing Pilates — Obliques (15-1)

How To?

1. Start from a kneeling position, with your hands behind your head. Now flex and rotate your trunk without losing axial elongation.
2. Return to the starting position, undoing the Twist and extending your trunk, until you reach a neutral spinal position.

Muscles Involved
- Rectus abdominis
- Minor oblique on the side of the Twist
- Major oblique on the side opposite the Twist
- Gluteus maximus
- Hamstrings

Main Stretch

Quadratus lumborum on the side opposite the Twist.

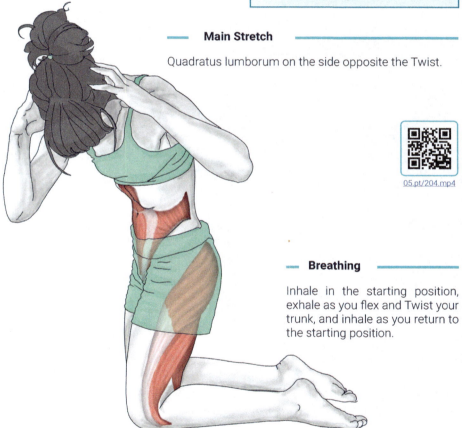

05.pt/204.mp4

Breathing

Inhale in the starting position, exhale as you flex and Twist your trunk, and inhale as you return to the starting position.

Differences and Similarities with the Floor Exercise

Since your base is smaller than in the floor exercise, this version will activate your obliques more strongly. However, the exercise is more aerial so you will need to pay concentrate harder on stabilizing your hips in order to feel the abdominal work fully. On the floor, the feeling of effort is immediate and easy to attain because you are working against gravity, but in the standing exercise the opposite is true.

Scissors (12-1)

Standing Pilates — 10

How To?

1. Start from a standing position with one leg raised and flexed and hands touching either side of your ankle.
2. Extend the flexed leg forward without losing hold of your ankle.

Muscles Involved

- Abdominal transverse
- Iliopsoas of the dynamic leg
- Quadriceps of the dynamic leg
- Glutes of the stabilizing leg
- Spinal erectors

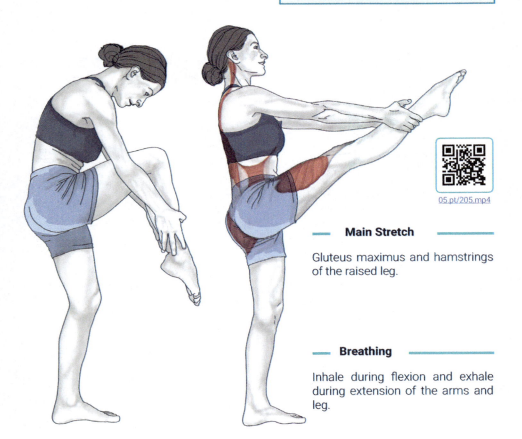

05.pt/205.mp4

Main Stretch

Gluteus maximus and hamstrings of the raised leg.

Breathing

Inhale during flexion and exhale during extension of the arms and leg.

Differences and Similarities with the Floor Exercise

In spite of the clear difference involved in keeping your balance, this exercise is actually very similar to its floor counterpart. It is more intense, however, because the lever formed by your leg must work against gravity, which requires more effort of the iliopsoas and quadriceps. Since there is no spinal flexion, the rectus abdominis acts as a stabilizer.

11 Standing Pilates — Prone Heel Squeeze (13-1)

How To?

1. Start from a standing position with your legs together and external rotation of the hips (toes pointing outward).
2. Flex your knees to a 90-degree angle, keeping the external hip rotation, and then return to the starting position.

Muscles Involved
- Adductors
- Lower fibers of the gluteus maximus
- Vastus medialis of the quadriceps

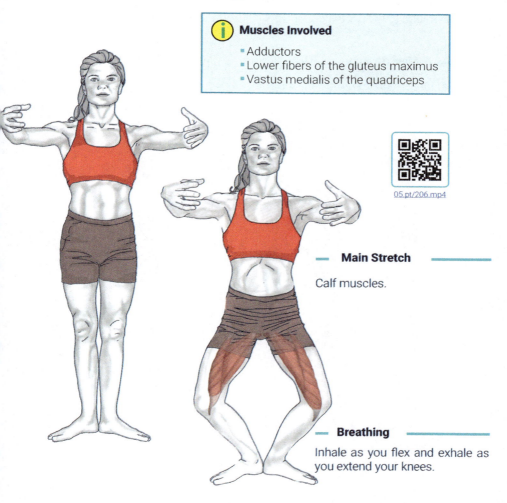

05.pt/206.mp4

Main Stretch

Calf muscles.

Breathing

Inhale as you flex and exhale as you extend your knees.

Differences and Similarities with the Floor Exercise

There is work here for all of the leg muscles, especially as you flex and extend your. It is far easier to keep your hips neutral when you are standing upright. Constraints in the descent are usually due to tight calf muscles. This is an excellent exercise to compensate for knock knees.

12 Standing Pilates — Saw (14-1)

How To?

1. Start from a standing position with your legs open and arms outstretched in a cross.
2. Rotate your trunk, allowing your arms and gaze to follow the movement, and then Twist to reach over to your opposite leg with your lower arm. Keep your hips neutral and facing forwards throughout.
3. Return to the neutral starting position, first undoing the Twist and then the spinal flexion.

Main Stretch

Quadratus lumborum on the side opposite the Twist.

Muscles Involved

- Major abdominal oblique on the side opposite the Twist.
- Minor abdominal oblique on the side of the Twist.

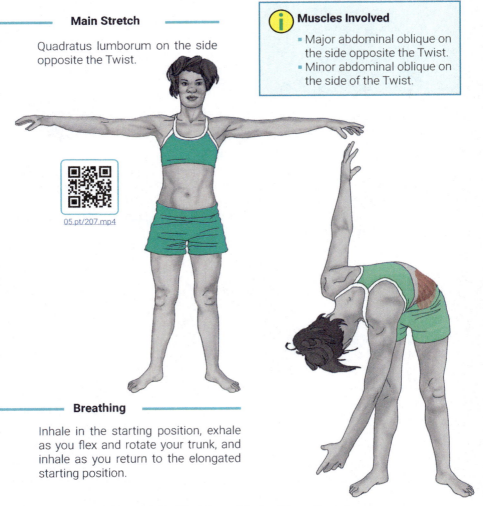

05.pt/207.mp4

Breathing

Inhale in the starting position, exhale as you flex and rotate your trunk, and inhale as you return to the elongated starting position.

Differences and Similarities with the Floor Exercise

These are very similar exercises once you realize that the power needed for the Twist and trunk flexion comes from the abdomen. If you do not bear this in mind, just another stretch.

13 Standing Pilates — Oblique Roll-Up (5-1)

How To?

1. Start from a standing position with your arms raised. Now flex and rotate your trunk without losing axial elongation.
2. To go back to the starting position, undo the Twist and extend your trunk until your spine returns to the neutral position.

Main Stretch

Quadratus lumborum on the side opposite the Twist.

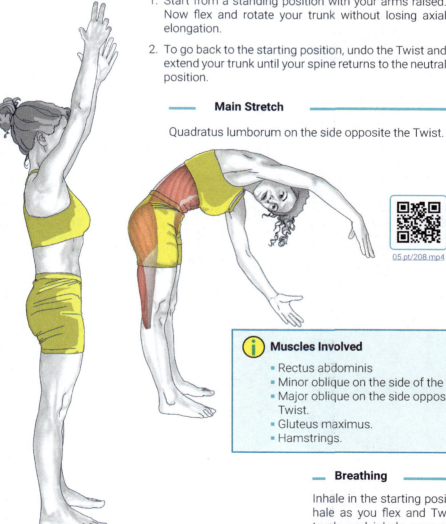

05.pt/208.mp4

Muscles Involved

- Rectus abdominis
- Minor oblique on the side of the Twist.
- Major oblique on the side opposite the Twist.
- Gluteus maximus.
- Hamstrings.

Breathing

Inhale in the starting position, exhale as you flex and Twist your trunk, and inhale once more as you return to the starting position.

Differences and Similarities with the Floor Exercise

Raising your arms means makes the lever formed by your trunk longer, which will increase the intensity of the exercise. The longer lever makes it easier to flex your trunk since you will have the aid of gravity. However, the difficulty increases when you keep on flexing so that and the force of gravity works to drag you towards the floor. This requires you to use hamstrings and glutes as a brake.

14 Standing Pilates — One Side Leg Kick (16-1)

How To?

1. Start from a standing position with the hand opposite to your working leg on your abdomen and the other arm outstretched.
2. Lift your leg sideways and away from your outstretched arm, keeping your knee facing forwards. 3. Bring your leg back to the starting position without touching the floor with your foot. This means you must flex your knee slightly.

Muscles Involved

- Gluteus medius and minor of the dynamic leg.
- Tensor fasciae latae of the dynamic leg.
- Pyramidalis of the dynamic leg.
- Deltoid glute of the balancing leg.

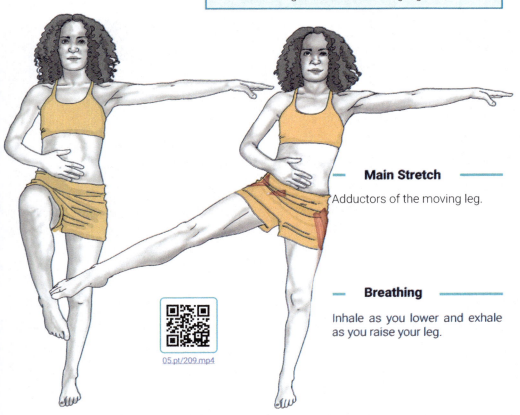

Main Stretch

Adductors of the moving leg.

Breathing

Inhale as you lower and exhale as you raise your leg.

05.pt/209.mp4

Differences and Similarities with the Floor Exercise

The muscle work of the moving leg is very similar. However, the other leg also has balance work to do, which is not the case in the floor exercise.

15 — Standing Pilates — Side Leg Series, Var. 3 (17-1)

How To?

1. Start from a standing position with the hand opposite to your working leg on your abdomen and the other arm outstretched.
2. Lift your leg sideways and away from your outstretched arm while keeping your knee facing forwards or rotating your hips outwards, depending on your goals.
3. Keep your leg motionless while you move your ankle to draw circles with your toes in both directions. You can also flex and extend your ankle.

Muscles Involved

- Gluteus medius and minor of the raised leg.
- Tensor fasciae latae of the raised leg.
- Pyramidalis of the raised leg. Calf muscles and anterior tibialis of the raised leg.
- Deltoid glute of the balancing leg.

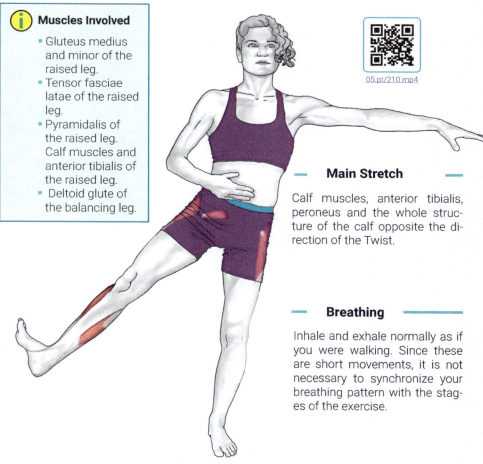

05.pt/210.mp4

Main Stretch

Calf muscles, anterior tibialis, peroneus and the whole structure of the calf opposite the direction of the Twist.

Breathing

Inhale and exhale normally as if you were walking. Since these are short movements, it is not necessary to synchronize your breathing pattern with the stages of the exercise.

Differences and Similarities with the Floor Exercise

This exercise is fairly similar to Variation 3 of the Side Leg Series, a Level 1 exercise. The muscle work of the dynamic leg is very similar, but the supporting leg also works to keep your balance, which is not the case in the floor exercise.

Single Leg Extension (20-1)

Standing Pilates

How To?

1. Start from a standing position with your arms extended forwards and one knee flexed and slightly raised.
2. Extend your leg backwards as you extend your hips, then do slight leg raises while keeping your hips neutral.

Muscles Involved

- Gluteus maximus of the raised leg.
- Superior fibers of the hamstrings of the raised leg.
- Abductors of the supporting leg.

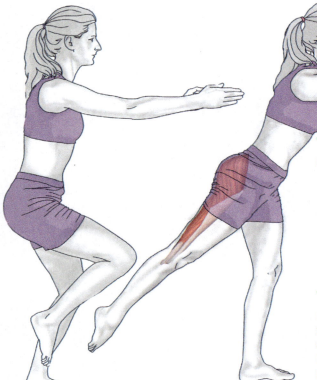

05.pt/211.mp4

Main Stretch

Iliopsoas of the raised leg.

Breathing

If you are making a broad movement, inhale during the flexion and exhale for each extension. If you keep your leg raised and pulse, breathe steadily as if you were walking.

Differences and Similarities with the Floor Exercise

Not having your hips on the floor allows you to raise your leg higher, which increases the workload for your glutes. However, you will need to concentrate on keeping your hips and trunk stable throughout the exercise. The supporting leg works in the same way as in other similar exercises, which is not the case in the floor exercise.

Shell Stretch (1-1)

Standing Pilates

How To?

1. Start from a standing position with a slight flexion of your knees and your arms on either side of your trunk.
2. Flex your trunk deeply, relaxing your head and arms to drop them in front of your trunk.

> **Muscles Involved**
> - Quadriceps.

Main Stretch

Quadratus lumborum and spinal erectors

05.pt/212.mp4

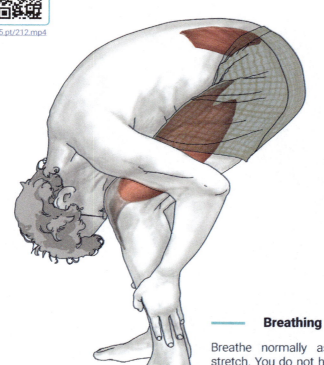

Breathing

Breathe normally as you hold the stretch. You do not have to follow any specific breathing pattern.

Differences and Similarities with the Floor Exercise

This is a more tonic exercise, because you have to hold the position on your two feet. However, there is a greater relaxation of the shoulders and cervical region.

18 Standing Pilates — Push up (14-2)

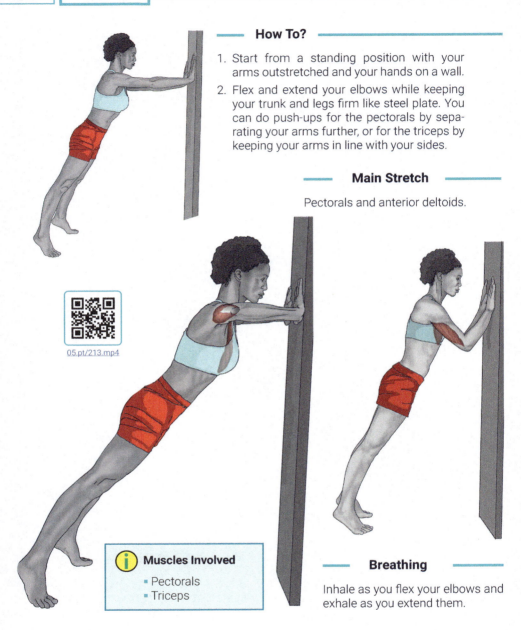

How To?

1. Start from a standing position with your arms outstretched and your hands on a wall.
2. Flex and extend your elbows while keeping your trunk and legs firm like steel plate. You can do push-ups for the pectorals by separating your arms further, or for the triceps by keeping your arms in line with your sides.

Main Stretch

Pectorals and anterior deltoids.

05.pt/213.mp4

Muscles Involved

- Pectorals
- Triceps

Breathing

Inhale as you flex your elbows and exhale as you extend them.

Differences and Similarities with the Floor Exercise

Wall push-ups are far less intense, and this exercise is therefore recommended as an initiation to floor push-ups.

19 Standing Pilates — Chair (without floor support)

How To?

1. Start from a standing position with your arms by your sides or extended forwards.
2. Flex your knees deeply, leaning your trunk forwards. Your knees should never come further forward than your feet and your back must stay elongated and neutral.

Muscles Involved
- Quadriceps
- Glutes

Main Stretch

Gluteus maximus

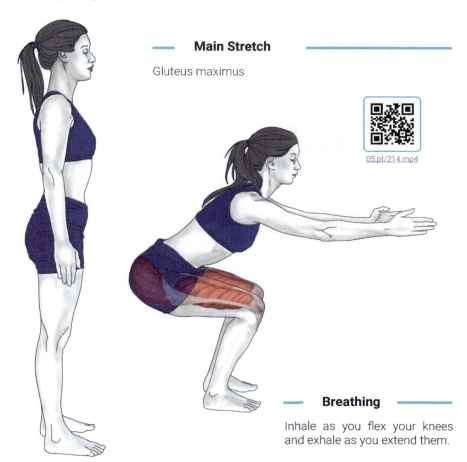

05.pt/214.mp4

Breathing

Inhale as you flex your knees and exhale as you extend them.

Differences and Similarities with the Floor Exercise

Because you need to keep your hips neutral, it is harder to attain a full abdominal workload. However, the need to keep the hips in place encourages work for glutes and hamstrings.

20 Standing Pilates — Split (Without Reference on the Floor)

How To?

1. Start from a standing position with your legs in a scissors position and your arms by your sides or outstretched forwards.
2. Flex your knees deeply, keeping the heel of your back leg raised throughout. The knee of the front leg should never come further forward than your foot.

Muscles Involved
- Quadriceps
- Glutes

Main Stretch

Gluteus maximus

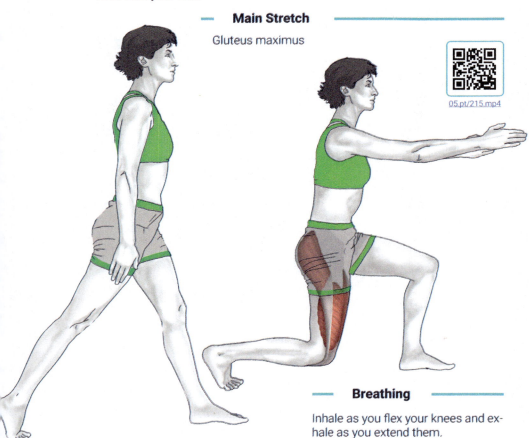

Breathing

Inhale as you flex your knees and exhale as you extend them.

Differences and Similarities with the Floor Exercise

Without pressure from the floor on your front, it is far easier to extend your spine. However, this easy way to do the exercise can be negative without proper pelvic stabilization.

21 — Standing Pilates — Oblique Split (Without floor support)

How To?

1. Start from a standing position with your legs in a scissors position and your arms by your sides or outstretched.
2. Flex your knees deeply, keeping the heel of your back leg raised throughout. The knee of the front leg should never come further forward than your foot.
3. Twist your trunk without moving your hips or legs. Undo the Twist and return to starting position.

Muscles Involved
- Quadriceps
- Glutes
- Major and Minor Obliques.

Main Stretch

Gluteus maximus and quadratus lumborum on the side opposite the Twist.

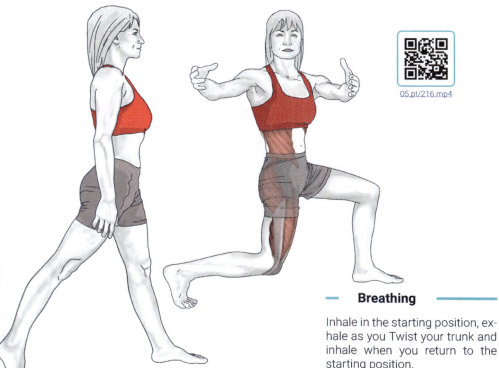

05.pt/216.mp4

Breathing

Inhale in the starting position, exhale as you Twist your trunk and inhale when you return to the starting position.

Differences and Similarities with the Floor Exercise

Inhale as you flex your knees and exhale as you Twist your trunk, then inhale as you undo the Twist and exhale as you return to the starting position.

22 Standing Pilates — Back and Forth (without floor support)

How To?

1. Start from a standing position with your arms by your sides.
2. Sway back and forth without separating your heels or toes from the floor. Keep your trunk and legs stiff like a plank.

Muscles Involved
- Calf muscles
- Anterior tibialis

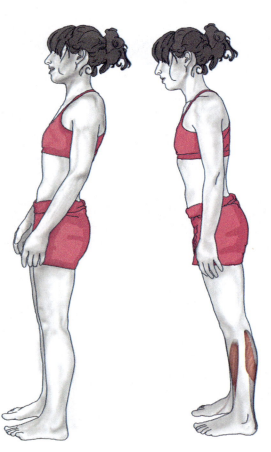

05.pt/217.mp4

Main Stretch

Calf Muscles

Breathing

You can decide when to inhale and when to exhale depending what you find most comfortable, since there is no stage of this exercise that is more intense than any other.

Differences and Similarities with the Floor Exercise

It is far easier to extend your spine without pressure from the floor on your front. However, this easier way of doing the exercise can be negative without proper pelvic stabilization.

23 Standing Pilates — Relevé (without floor support)

How To?

1. Start from a standing position with your arms by your sides.
2. Stand on tiptoes (plantar flexion of the ankles) while raising your arms as if you were a torpedo, at the same time trying to touch the ceiling with the crown of your head.

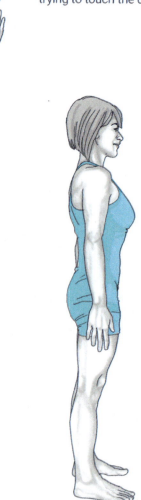

Muscles Involved
- Calf Muscles

Main Stretch

Anterior tibialis

Breathing

Exhale during ascent, inhale during descent.

Differences and Similarities with the Floor Exercise

Because you need to keep your hips neutral it will be more difficult to do the full abdominal work. However, the need to keep your hips neutral works your glutes and hamstrings.

Standing Pilates — One Leg Kick (4-2)

How To?

1. From a standing position, with arms outstretched forwards and one of your legs extended backwards.
2. Flex your knee, bringing your heel up towards your butt without lowering your leg.

Muscles Involved

- Gluteus maximus of the raised leg.
- Upper fibers of the hamstrings of the raised leg.
- Quadriceps and hip muscles of the supporting leg.

Main Stretch

Iliopsoas of the working leg.

Quadriceps of the working leg.

Breathing

Exhale as you flex your knee, and inhale as you extend it.

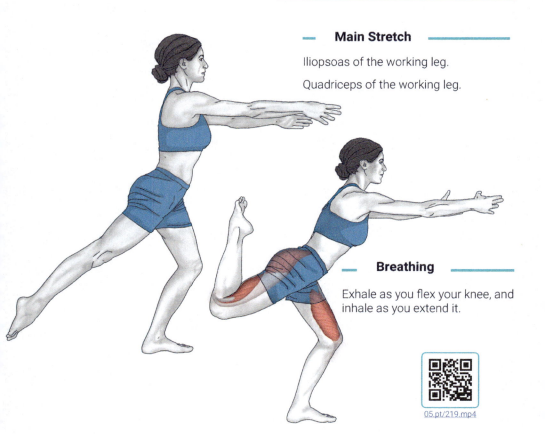

05.pt/219.mp4

Differences and Similarities with the Floor Exercise

The leg is not raised in the floor exercise, so there is no extension of the hips, which remain in a neutral position. This can also be done standing, if you can manage to extend your leg as an extension of your trunk. The exercise improves proprioception of the neutral hips in a situation without any support point. The transference from this exercise to everyday activities is highly beneficial.

Swimming Arms (10-2)

Standing Pilates — 25

How To?

1. Start from a kneeling position with arms raised.
2. Flex one shoulder and then other alternately, stretching back behind your head if your joint mobility allows you to.

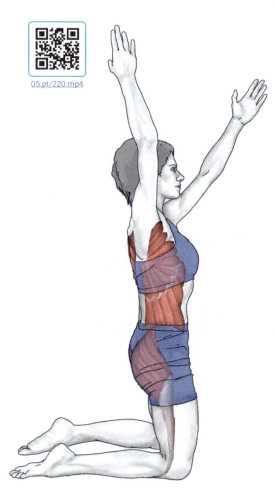

05.pt/220.mp4

Muscles Involved

- Abdominal obliques
- Serrate
- Trapezius
- Glutes

Main Stretch

Latissimus dorsi

Breathing

Inhale in the starting position and continue by breathing to the rhythm of the motion of your arms in a steady harmonious pattern, as if you were walking.

Differences and Similarities with the Floor Exercise

Since the position is freer, your ribcage is less likely to close, allowing for a longer movement of the arms. However, this is a mistake that will turn the exercise into something very different from the goals of the Pilates Method.

Side Bend (13-2)

Standing Pilates — 26

How To?

1. Start from a standing position, with your knees semi-flexed, hands resting on your shins and spine flexed.
2. Step sideways with one leg (abduction), moving it away from your center, as you stretch out your arm, trunk and other leg.
3. Return to the starting position in in a harmonious movement flow, as if you were floating. First flex the extended leg, then do a squat and approach with the working leg.

Muscles Involved

- Quadriceps
- Adductors
- Abdominal obliques

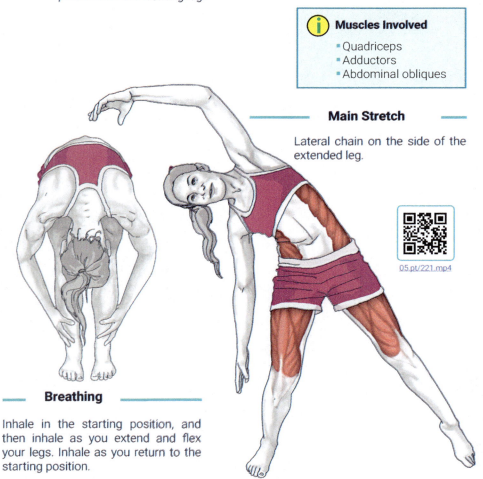

Main Stretch

Lateral chain on the side of the extended leg.

05.pt/221.mp4

Breathing

Inhale in the starting position, and then inhale as you extend and flex your legs. Inhale as you return to the starting position.

Differences and Similarities with the Floor Exercise

The strength work now belongs to the muscles of the lower body and the stretches to the upper body. However, this exercise fully stretches the whole lateral chains, alternating between sides.

27 Standing Pilates — Swimming (10-2)

How To?

1. Start from a standing position with knees semi-flexed and arms raised.
2. Raise the hip and knee of one leg and draw the opposite arm back.
3. Repeat with the other arm and leg, keeping your knees semi-flexed throughout.

Muscles Involved

- Glutes
- Trapezius
- Rhomboids
- Abdominal obliques

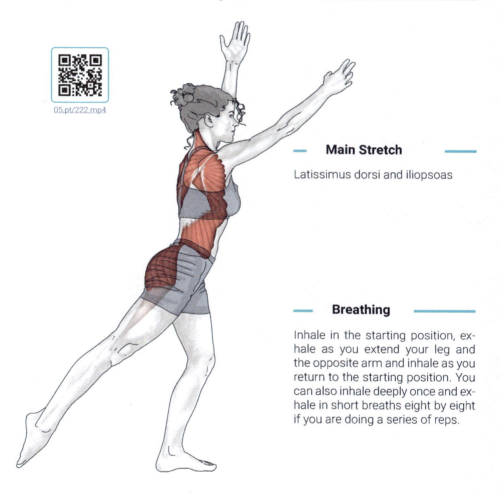

05.pt/222.mp4

Main Stretch

Latissimus dorsi and iliopsoas

Breathing

Inhale in the starting position, exhale as you extend your leg and the opposite arm and inhale as you return to the starting position. You can also inhale deeply once and exhale in short breaths eight by eight if you are doing a series of reps.

Differences and Similarities with the Floor Exercise

Since the hips are not supported the floor, the work of pelvic stabilization is far more conscious in this exercise. However, this is a good option for those who cannot do the swimming exercise on the floor for lack of shoulder mobility.

28 Standing Pilates — Triceps Kick (Lower Body)

How To?

1. Kneel with knees flexed at an angle above 90 degrees, hips flexed and arms by your side with your spine elongated and trunk leaning forwards.
2. Extend your elbows back without moving your upper arm from its original position. If you raise and lower your whole arm, you will cease to feel the work of your triceps.

  Muscles Involved
- Triceps
- Posterior deltoids
- Quadriceps

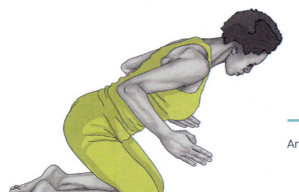

05.pt/223.mp4

Main Stretch

Anterior deltoids and pectorals.

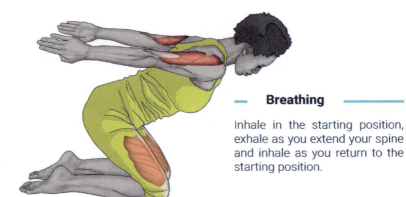

Breathing

Inhale in the starting position, exhale as you extend your spine and inhale as you return to the starting position.

Differences and Similarities with the Floor Exercise

Inhale as you flex your elbows and exhale as you extend them, drawing deep and slow breaths.

Tables of Exercises by Goal

Tables of Exercises by Goal

This chapter contains a careful selection of exercises grouped into ten tables, which can be done in a very short time yet provide great benefits. The exercises are designed:

- To strengthen and reduce the abdomen
- To increase energy
- To increase energy
- To improve everyday agility
- For the shoulders, back and chest
- For the glutes, hips, and legs
- To improve joint mobility
- For back care
- For bedtime
- For a pleasant morning routine

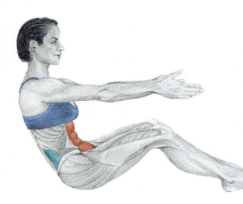

You will not always have time to do a full workout. In these cases, my suggestion is that you exercise more consciously, listening to your body in order decide what you need in the moment. Then choose the right table.

You must apply the principles of the method in each exercise and ensure you do them with good form. Never forget that the key is not doing the exercise but how you do it.

To strengthen and reduce the abdomen

Work for the four groups of abdominal muscles (rectus abdominis, major and minor obliques and abdominal transverse) through concentric, eccentric and isometric contractions.

Half Roll Back

Exercise 4, Level 1
Routine: 2 series of 8 repetitions, resting between series.

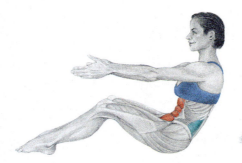

Ab Prep

Exercise 1, Level 1
Routine: 2 blocks made up of 3 series of 8 repetitions, resting between blocks.

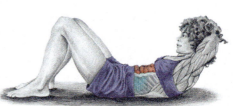

Squad

Exercise 25, Level 1
Routine: 2 blocks made up of 3 series of 8 repetitions, resting between blocks.

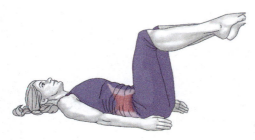

Roll over

Exercise 3, Level 2
Routine: 1 series of 8 repetitions done slowly

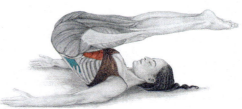

To strengthen and reduce the abdomen

Half Roll Back Obliques
Exercise 15, Level 1
Routine: 2 series of 8 repetitions.

Teaser series
Exercise 2, Level 3
Routine: 1 series of 8 repetitions of each variation.

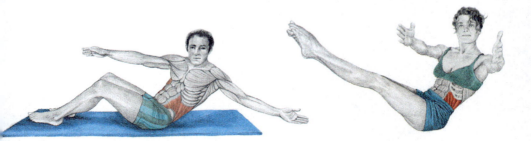

Leg Pull Front
Exercise 11, Level 2
Routine: 1 series of 8 repetitions done slowly.

Cat and Horse
Exercise 23, Level 1
Routine: 1 series of 8 repetitions done slowly.

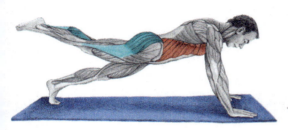
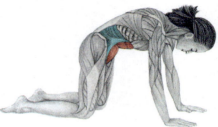

To strengthen and reduce the abdomen

Trunk Rotation Stretch

Exercise 24, Level 1

Routine: One minute of passive relaxation and stretching, allowing you to rest your legs on the floor.

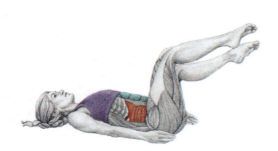

Supine Shell Stretch

Exercise 22, Level 1

Routine: One minute of passive relaxation and stretching.

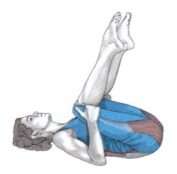

To increase energy

A combination of strength and flexibility exercises for different muscle groups with proper breathing.

Hundred

Exercise 3, Level 1

Routine: Do Variation 1 of the exercise once.

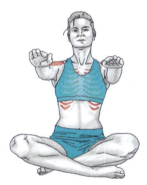

Half Roll Back

Exercise 4, Level 1

Routine: 2 series of 8 repetitions with backward inclination but without full elevation, resting between series.

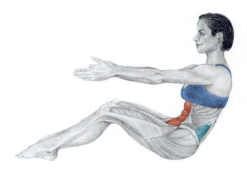

Abdominal Series

Exercise 26, Level 1

Routine: 1 series of 8 repetitions done of each variation.

One Foot Circles

Exercise 17, Level 1

Routine: 3 series of 8 repetitions per side and foot.

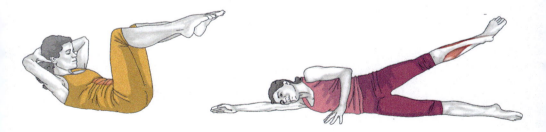

To increase energy

Cat and Horse
Exercise 23, Level 1

Routine: 1 series of 8 repetitions done slowly.

Breast Stroke
Exercise 2, Level 1

Routine: 2 series of 8 repetitions, resting between series.

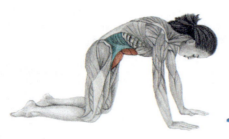
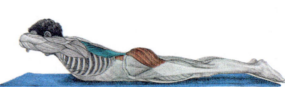

Shell Stretch
Exercise 22, Level 1

Routine: One minute of active relax and stretch, Variation 1.

Side Bend
Exercise 13, Level 2

Routine: 6 repetitions per side.

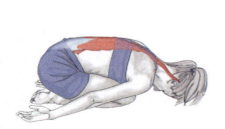
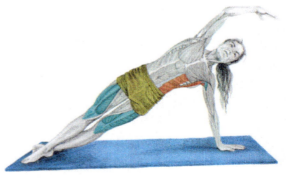

To increase energy

Trunk Rotation
Exercise 24, Level 1

Routine: 2 series of 8 repetitions, resting between series.

Roll Like a Ball
Exercise 8, Level 1

Routine: 1 series of 8 repetitions.

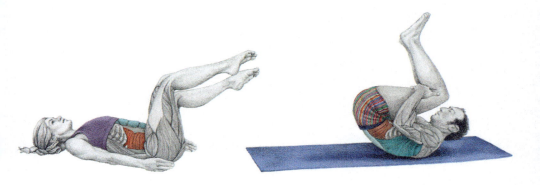

Use whatever you have at hand in the workplace. Chairs, desks and walls can become a training facility.

Cat and Horse
Exercise 23, Level 1

Routine: 1 series of 8 repetitions done slowly. Variation 2, sitting on a chair.

Chair
Exercise 20, Standing Exercises.

Routine: 2 blocks of 3 series of 8 repetitions. Done on a chair.

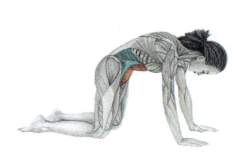
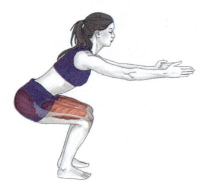

For the work place

Push-Up

Exercise 18, Standing Exercises.

Routine: 2 blocks of 2 series of 8 repetitions. Done on a desk.

Triceps Kick

Exercise 28, de Standing Exercises.

Routine: 2 series of 8 repetitions. Variation 2, done on a chair.

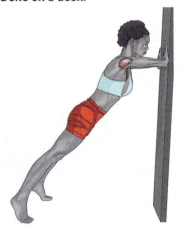
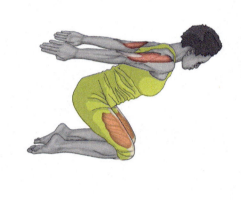

One Leg Kick

Exercise 25, Standing Exercises.

Routine: 2 blocks made up of 3 series of 8 repetitions, with support on a table or wall.

One Side Leg Kick

Exercise 14, Standing Exercises.

Routine: 3 series of 8 repetitions, with support on a table or wall.

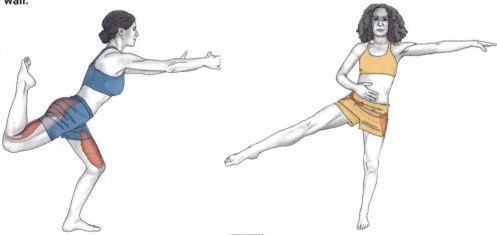

For the work place

Ab Prep

Exercise 1, Standing Exercises.

Routine: 2 blocks made up of 3 series of 8 repetitions, sitting on a chair.

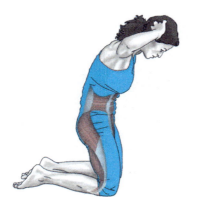

Breast Stroke

Exercise 2, Standing Exercises.

Routine: 2 series of 8 repetitions, sitting on a chair.

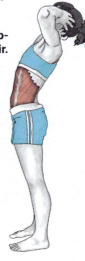

Side Bend

Exercise 28, Standing Exercises.

Routine: 1 series of 8 repetitions.

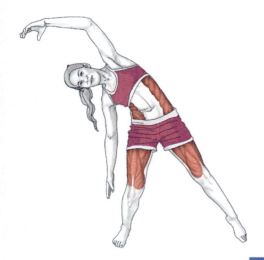

Shell Stretch

Exercise 17, Standing Exercises.

Routine: Hold the position for 20 seconds. Repeat 2 times.

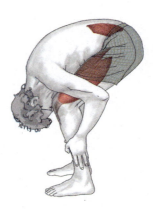

For the work place

The mermaid
Exercise number 28, standing pilates.

Routine: 1 serie of 8 repetitions.

Child's pose
Exercise number 17, standing pilates.

Routine: hold the posture for 20 seconds, repeat it twice.

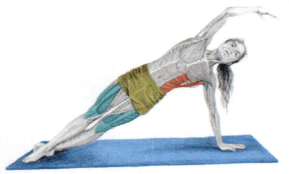
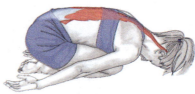

To improve everyday agility

This group of exercises to train joint mobility and muscle strength. It includes standing exercises as a key part of transference to everyday activities.

Three-Time Breathing

Exercise 7 of the Breathing principle.

Routine: 1 series of 8 repetitions.

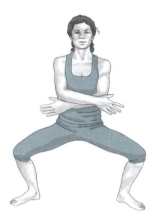

Spinal Articulation in Standing Position

Exercise 3 of the Axial Elongation principle.

Routine: 1 series of 8 repetitions.

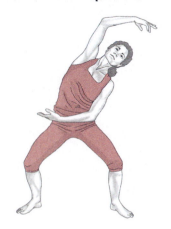

Roll Like a Ball

Exercise 8, Level 1.

Routine: 1 series of 8 repetitions.

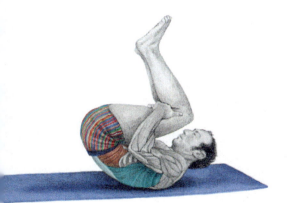

Posterior Breathing

Exercise 3 of the Breathing principle.

Routine: 1 series of 8 repetitions.

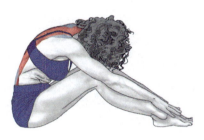

To improve everyday agility

Twist

Exercise 7, Level 1.

Routine: 2 series of 8 repetitions.

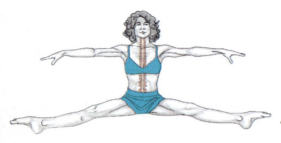

Roll up

Exercise 5, Level 1.

Routine: 1 series of 8 repetitions.

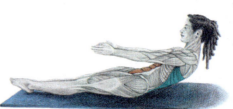

Saw

Exercise 14, Level 1.

Routine: 1 series of 8 repetitions.

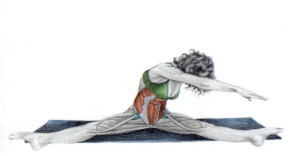

Bridge

Exercise 2, Level 2.

Routine: 2 blocks made up of 2 series of 4 repetitions. Variation 1.

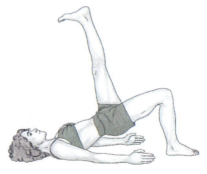

To improve everyday agility

Breast Stroke
Exercise 2, Level 1.

Routine: 1 series of 8 repetitions. Variation.

Push up
Exercise 14, Level 2.

Routine: 1 series of 4 repetitions. Variation 2.

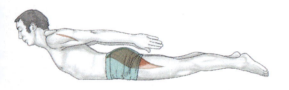
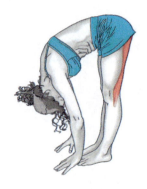

For the shoulders, back and chest

Work for the upper body, combining exercises of different levels. The most advanced exercises can be modified to lower the difficulty (see Variations).

Cross

Exercise 6 of the Scapular Stabilization Principle

Routine: 3 series of one minute each holding the stretch position.

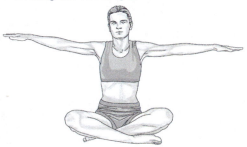

Swimming

Exercise 10, Level 2.

Routine: 2 series of 8 repetitions in slow motion.

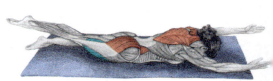

Leg Pull

Exercise 10, Level 2.

Routine: 2 series of 8 repetitions in slow motion.

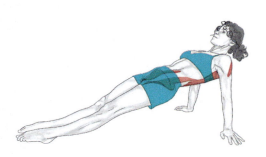

Push-Ups

Exercise 14, Position 4, Level 2

Routine: 3 series of 4 push-ups.

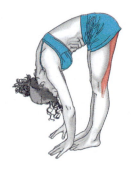

For the shoulders, back and chest

Half Roll Back Obliques
Exercise 15, Level 1.

Routine: 2 series de 8 repetitions.

Jackknife
Exercise 7, Level 2.

Routine: 1 series of 4 repetitions.

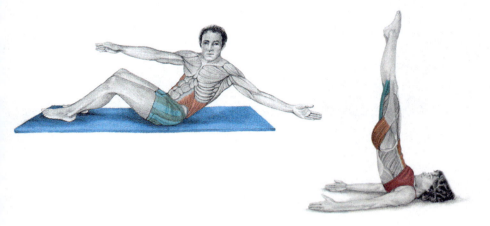

Side Bend
Exercise 13, Level 2.

Routine: 1 series of 6 repetitions per side.

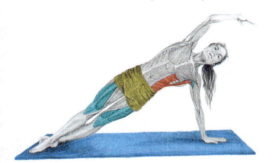

Leg Pull
Exercise 4, Level 3. Variation 1.

Routine: 1 series of 8 repetitions per leg.

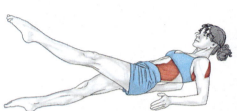

For the shoulders, back and chest

Shell Stretch
Exercise 22, Level 1.

Routine: One minute.

Anterior Chain Stretch
Exercise 7E, basic stretch positions.

Routine: One minute.

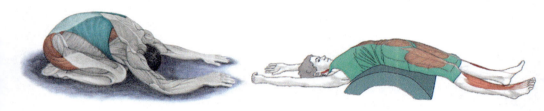

For the glutes, hips, and legs

Lower body workout, combining exercises of different levels to develop and train endurance and muscle tone.

Split

Exercise 20, Standing

Routine: 2 blocks made up of 2 series of 8 repetitions per leg.

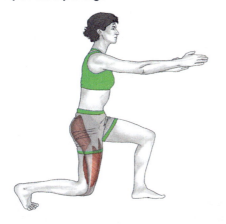

Prone Glute

Exercise 20, Level 1.

Routine: 2 series de 8 repetitions. Variation 1.

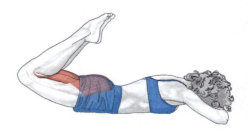

Bridge

Exercise 2, Level 2.

Routine: 2 series of 8 repetitions, with legs together.

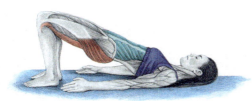

Side Leg Series

Exercise 17, Level 1.

Routine: 4 series of 8 repetitions per leg.

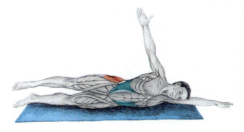

For the glutes, hips, and legs

Squad

Exercise 25, Level 1.

Routine: 2 blocks of 3 series of 8 repetitions.

One Leg Stretch

Exercise 8, Standing Exercises.

Routine: 2 blocks made up of 1 series of 4 repetitions per leg.

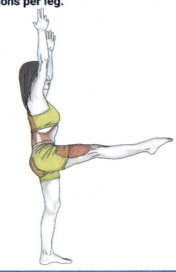

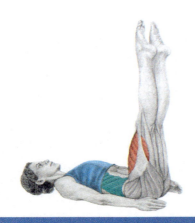

Hinge

Exercise 15, Level 2.

Routine: 2 blocks made up of 2 series of 8 repetitions.

Side Kick Kneeling

Exercise 3, Level 3.

Routine: 2 blocks made up of 1 series of 8 repetitions on each leg.

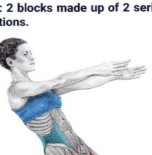

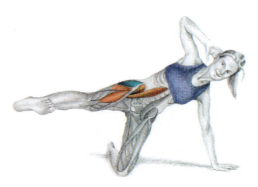

For the glutes, hips, and legs

Quadriceps Stretch

Exercise 1E, basic stretch positions.

Routine: One minute per leg.

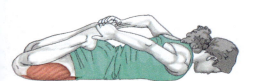

Hamstring Stretch

Exercise 2E, basic stretch positions.

Routine: One minute per leg.

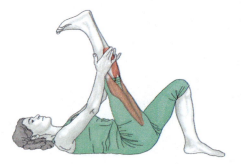

To improve joint mobility

Easy mobility exercises to keep your joints healthy and improve your range of movement.

Scapular Abduction/Adduction

Exercise 1, Scapular Stabilization principle

Routine: 2 series of 8 repetitions.

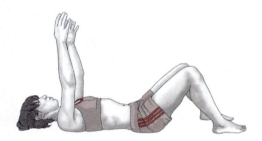

Pelvic Anteversion/Retroversion

Exercise 1, Pelvic Stabilization principle

Routine: 2 series of 8 repetitions.

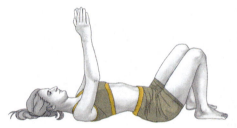

Bridge

Exercise 2, Level 2

Routine: 2 series of 8 repetitions

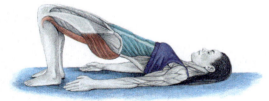

Hip twist

Exercise 5, Pelvic Stabilization principle

Routine: 1 series of 8 repetitions per leg.

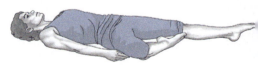

To improve joint mobility

Roll up
Exercise 5, Level 1.

Routine: 1 series of 8 repetitions.

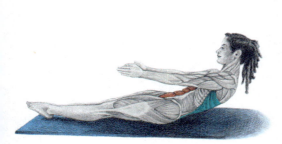

Slow Double Leg Stretch
Exercise 1, Level 2.

Routine: 1 series of 8 repetitions.

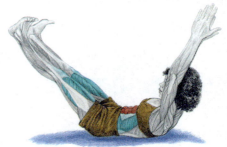

Flexo-Extension of the Ankles
Exercise 25, Level 1, Variation 4.

Routine: 3 series de 8 repetitions.

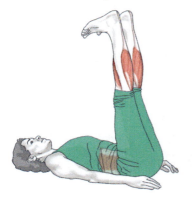

Trunk Rotation
Exercise 24, Level 1.

Routine: 2 series de 8 repetitions.

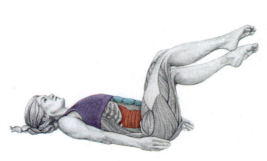

To improve joint mobility

Anterior Chain Stretch
Exercise 7 E.

Routine: One minute.

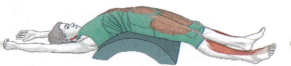

Posterior Chain Stretch
Exercise 8

Routine: One minute.

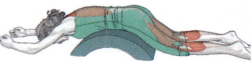

For back care

Abdominal and lower back strength exercises, mixed with stretches and spinal mobilization exercises to develop and maintain a strong, healthy back.

Dynamic Posterior Breathing

Exercise 1 of the Breathing principle.

Routine: 2 minutes of mobilization and slow breathing.

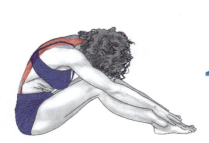

Breast Stroke

Exercise 2, Level 1.

Routine: 2 series de 8 repetitions.

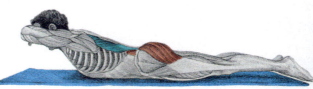

Ab Prep

Exercise 1, Level 1.

Routine: 3 series of 8 repetitions. Do 2 blocks if you are strong enough.

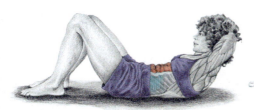

Saw

Exercise 14, Level 1.

Routine: 2 series de 8 repetitions.

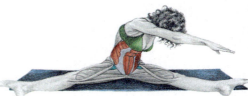

For back care

Side Leg Series

Exercise 17, Level 1.

Routine: 3 series of 8 repetitions per leg. You can choose either the basic exercise or any of the variations, or combine them in different patterns.

Spinal Articulation

Exercise 2 of the Axial Elongation principle.

Routine: 2 series of 8 repetitions.

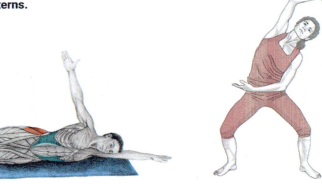

Pelvic Anteversion/Retroversion

Exercise 1, Pelvic Stabilization principle

Routine: 2 series of 8 repetitions.

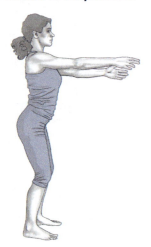

Prone Glute

Exercise 27, Level 1, Variation 1.

Routine: 3 series of 8 repetitions per leg.

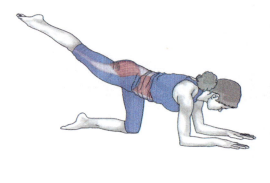

For back care

Cat and Horse: Muslim Prayer version

Exercise 23, Level 1, Variation 2.

Routine: 1 series of 4 repetitions.

Shell Stretch

Exercise 22, Level 1, Variation 1.

Routine: 2 minutes.

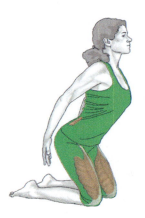
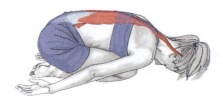

For bedtime

Articular mobilization, gentle activation and stretch of some muscle groups, and relaxing stretches to prepare your body and mind for sleep.

Hip twist

Exercise 5, Pelvic Stabilization principle

Routine: 1 series of 8 repetitions per leg.

Trunk Rotation

Exercise 24, Level 1.

Routine: 1 series of 8 repetitions.

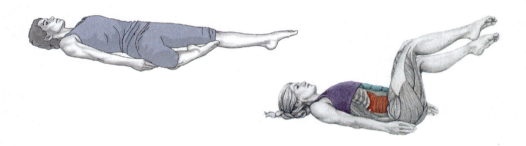

Upper Glute and Lower Back Stretch

Exercise 3E of "Stretches"

Routine: Hold the position for 30 seconds.

Squad

Exercise 25, Level 1.

Routine: 2 series of 8 repetitions.

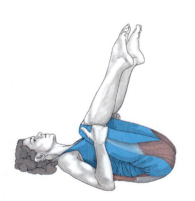
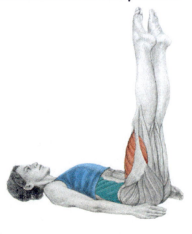

For bedtime

Quadriceps Stretch

Exercise 1E, from "Stretches"

Routine: Hold the position for 30 seconds per leg.

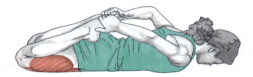

Side and Glutes Stretch

Exercise 4E, from "Stretches"

Routine: Hold the position for 1 minute per leg.

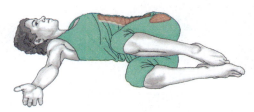

Dorsal Stretch

Exercise 5E, from "Stretches"

Routine: Hold the position for 1 minute.

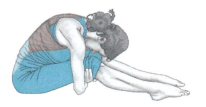

Lateral Chain Stretchlateral

Exercise 9E, from "Stretches"

Routine: Hold the position for one minute on each side.

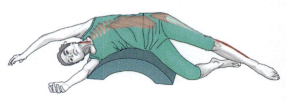

For bedtime

Neck Stretch

Exercise 12E, from "Stretches"

Routine: Hold each position for 20 seconds position. Do all the variations.

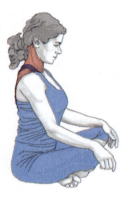

Breathing

Exercise 2, Breathing principle

Routine: 2 minutes of slow, deep, steady breathing.

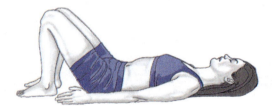

For a pleasant morning routine

Charge yourself up with healthy energy from the moment you get out of bed with mobilization and strength exercises for your main joints and muscle groups.

Pelvic Anteversion/Retroversion

Exercise 1, Pelvic Stabilization principle

Routine: 2 series of 8 repetitions.

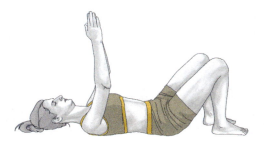

Trunk Flexion

Exercise 1, Axial Elongation principle

Routine: Hold the position for 30 seconds.

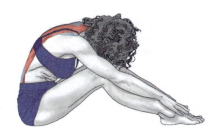

Cat and Horse

Exercise 14, Level 1.

Routine: Hold the position for 30 seconds.

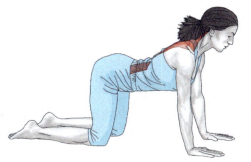

Ab Prep

Exercise 1, Level 1.

Routine: 2 series of 8 repetitions.

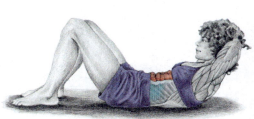

For a pleasant morning routine

One-Leg Circles

Exercise 6, Level 1.

Routine: 2 series of 8 circles per leg, in both directions: 2 series of 8 circles per leg, in both directions.

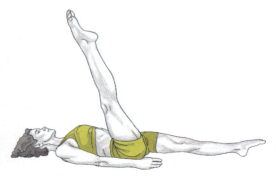

Saw

Exercise 14, Level 1. Variation with pelvic flexion.

Routine: 4 slow deep repetitions per side.

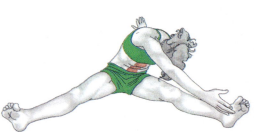

Axial Flexion

Exercise 19, Level 1

Routine: One series of 8 repetitions.

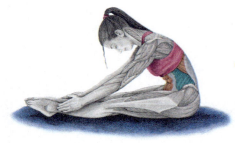

Prone Glute

Exercise 27, Level 1

Routine: 2 series of 8 repetitions per leg.

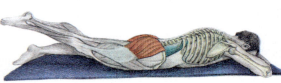

For a pleasant morning routine

Shell Stretch

Exercise 22, Level 1

Routine: Hold the position for 30 seconds.

Hundred

Exercise 3, Level 1. Variation 1.

Routine: One complete hundred flow. Exercise 3, Level 1. Variation 1.

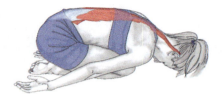
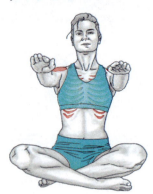

Masterclass

05.pt/masterclass7.mp4

To strengthen and reduce the abdomen

05.pt/masterclass9.mp4

To increase energy

05.pt/masterclass2.mp4

For the workplace

05.pt/masterclass6.mp4

To improve everyday agility

05.pt/masterclass10.mp4

For the shoulders, back and chest

05.pt/masterclass3.mp4

For the glutes, hips, and legs

05.pt/masterclass8.mp4

To improve joint mobility

05.pt/masterclass4.mp4

For back care

05.pt/masterclass1.mp4

For bedtime

05.pt/masterclass5.mp4

For a pleasant morning routine

Adaptations of exercises to frequent pathologies

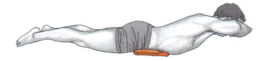

How to Use this Guide

Look for the challenge you face and solve it by applying the right adaptation. This chapter gathers together the commonest adaptations. Depending on the condition or weakness you suffer from or face, you may not be able to do some Level 3 exercises. However, there is no need to worry because the Pilates method offers numerous exercises to reap a broad spectrum of benefits and results without the need to reach an advanced level.

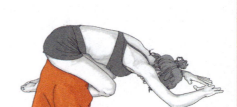

In this chapter, you will find some exercises that require similar and even interchangeable adaptations. For instance, "Leg Pull Front with Flexed Knees" is equally recommended for knee pain, hip pain and curvature of the spine (scoliosis). The goal in this case is to shorten the lever of your legs so as to ease the tension in the joints of your knees, hips and back.

Every exercise in this book includes adaptations with references that can be found in the list of adaptations, although you may also decide which adaptation to use knowing the constraints and/or pathologies affecting you or your students.

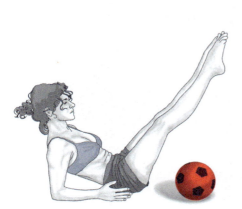

Common Adaptations

The Pilates method is appropriate for everyone, no matter their physical fitness or possible medical conditions that could constrain the exercises they can do. This means that constraints are not the problem in practice, but a challenge for the practitioner.

The following pages present a guide to the possibilities available to address constraints without having to skip the original Pilates exercises, or at least to be able to learn and do most of them. This goal can be attained with some very simple adaptations and easily available equipment.

Cushion	Mat

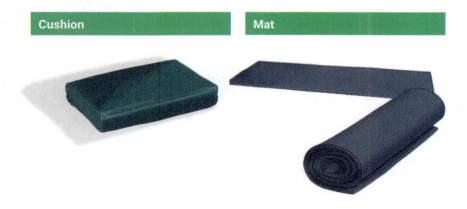

Arc

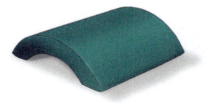

Roll

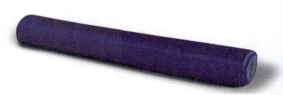

Resistance Band

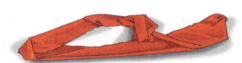

Ring

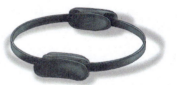

Foam Ball

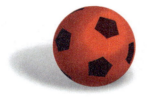

Bosu

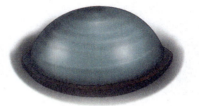

Index of adaptations

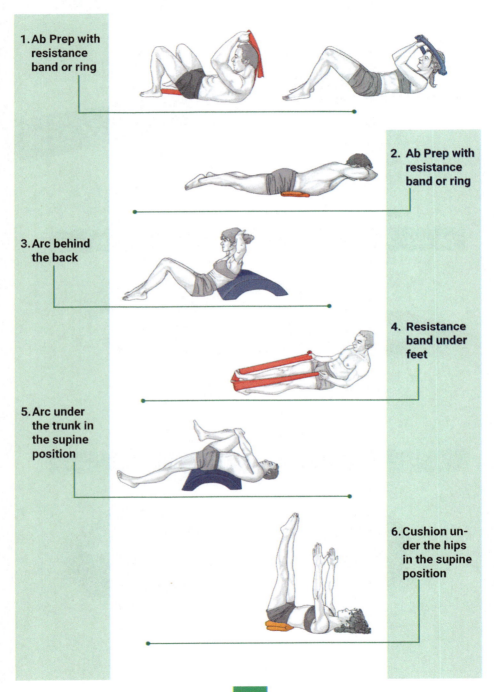

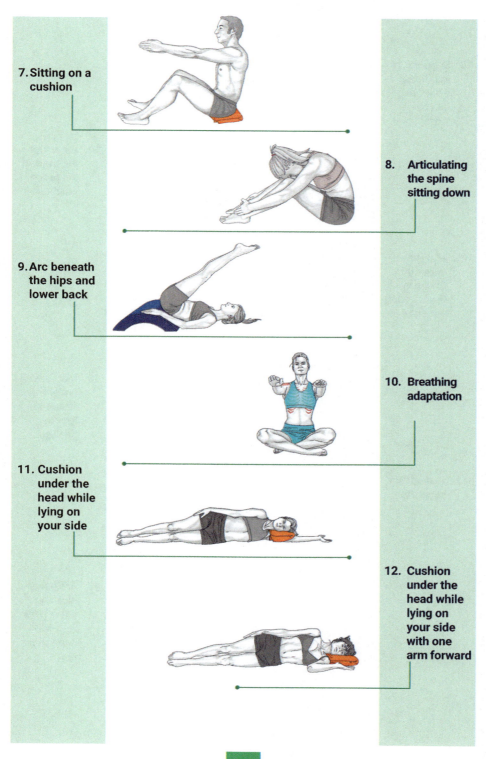

7. Sitting on a cushion
8. Articulating the spine sitting down
9. Arc beneath the hips and lower back
10. Breathing adaptation
11. Cushion under the head while lying on your side
12. Cushion under the head while lying on your side with one arm forward

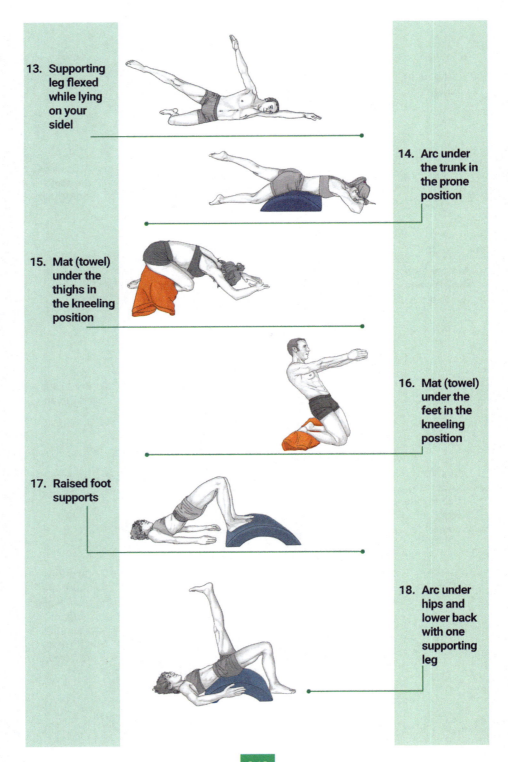

13. Supporting leg flexed while lying on your side!

14. Arc under the trunk in the prone position

15. Mat (towel) under the thighs in the kneeling position

16. Mat (towel) under the feet in the kneeling position

17. Raised foot supports

18. Arc under hips and lower back with one supporting leg

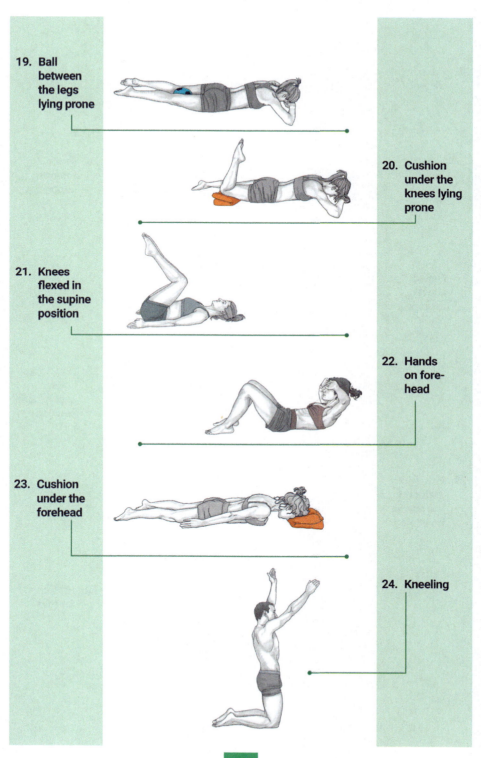

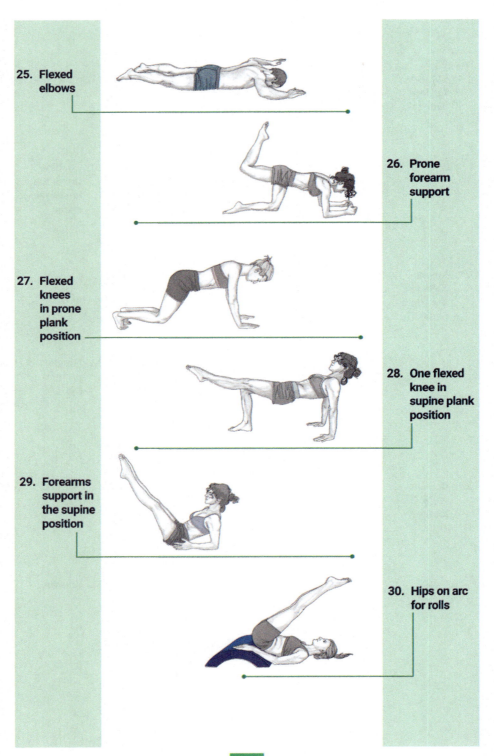

Adapted Exercises

Tightness

1. Sitting on a cushion, no. 7

To make the sitting position easier when the posterior muscle chains are tight, especially in the region of the hamstrings and glutes, and in the upper and lower back.

— Use a cushion if you find it hard to keep your spine elongated in upper body exercises using small devices (e.g. pectoral press with ring, hundred sitting down, articular mobilization of the shoulders, stretches of the neck muscles, and so forth).

2. Arc under the trunk in the supine lying position, no. 5

An initial stretch of the iliopsoas will reduce strain in exercises requiring pelvic extension.

— This should generally be done before you start exercises, especially those that require you to lie face down in a prone position, like the single leg extension, leg pull front, swimming, and so on.

3. Cushion under the hips in the supine position, no. 6

To eliminate lower back tension in case of tight muscles in the posterior chains or abdominal weakness.

— The cushion is used in exercises like two-leg circles and the corkscrew, among others, where the student is lying face up and the position of the legs produces excessive lordosis in the lower back.

4. Hips on arc for rolls, no. 29

Just like the cushion beneath the hips, the arc is used to eliminate lower back tension in case of tight posterior chain muscles or abdominal weakness.

— It is recommended for exercises involving pelvic flexion, spinal articulation, and approaching the legs to the trunk, such as roll over, jackknife, scissors in air, and so on.

5. Knees flexed in the supine position, no. 20

Sometimes no devices are needed to assist elevation of the legs without risk for the lower back, or the extension of the legs in sitting exercises: you only need to flex your knees in order to shorten the lever, allowing you to reduce the effort required to counteract gravity and stretch your muscle chains.

—You can do this in any exercise where you clearly cannot extend your knees without risk or without impeding spinal elongation.

Adductors/Open Legs

6. Ball between legs lying prone, number 18/19

People with strong abductor muscles often find that their open too far in exercises where the legs should be no more than hip-width apart. In this case, the constraint of keeping the ball in place keeps the adductor muscles active.

— Recommended for any exercise in which the principle of knees-hip alignment is essential, e.g. dorsal extension, ab prep, roll-up and others.

Neck muscles

7. Ab Prep with resistance band, no. 1

Just like home gyms for doing ab prep, but more economical. The resistance band keeps the head in place and the back of the neck still while eliminating the typical tension in the neck found when the technique has not yet been mastered. For the effect to be positive, you need to keep the band tight against your skull and motionless, thumbs glued to your forehead.

— This adaptation can be used in the Ab Prep and arms-free version of the Hundred exercises, and in all abdominal variations for the upper body.

8. Ab Prep with ring, no. 1

Similar to using a resistance band. The skull is placed against one of the ring's supports and both hands on the other support you place your hands, with the elbows flexed and shoulder-width apart. You have to exert pressure with your hands against the support and let the weight of the head rest against the ring.'

— For easy abdominal upper-body exercises.

9. Arc behind back, no. 3

Using an arc eliminates cervical strain by correcting the position of the neck, which becomes very similar to its position when standing.

— This adaptation may be used in exercises in which the trunk must be kept flexed, such as the hundred. It is also used in exercises with backwards trunk rolls to prevent the student from falling back completely, and in all the abdominal variations for the upper and lower body, when the support is placed a little nearer the neck and with the hands behind it.

10. Resistance band under the feet, no. 4

This reduces the effort required to counteract gravity, which makes it appropriate to reduce the work done by the lower back and to ensure proper positioning of the neck.

— The band can be used in of the half roll back and roll-up, exercises with raised legs, and so on, in which it will protect your back if your abdomen is still not strong enough to handle all of the workload. It is also recommended for the menstrual period, certain stages of pregnancy and in cases of chronic lower back pain and disc problems.

11. Prone forearm support, no. 26/28

The adaptation is used to eliminate support on the wrists in cases of chronic pain. It can also be used in case of cervical strain, but only if the student can achieve a good flexion of the spine.

— Prone forearm support can be used in leg pulls, mixed abdominals supported on the hands and to work the abdominal transverse muscles with your legs raised diagonally, as well as in the side bend and in its lateral abdominal variation.

Feet

12. Mat (towel) under the feet in the kneeling position, no. 15

Using a mat or folded towel will increase comfort in exercises involving the kneeling position for students who have little or no flexibility in their ankle joints.

– This adaptation is mainly used in the hinge and all of its variations, and in any other exercise which requires support on the front of your feet. The mat produces a slight flexion of the ankles, which is enough to reduce the articular strain that is sometimes the only reason why a practitioner cannot do this kind of exercises.

13. Supporting leg flexed lying on one's side, no. 12/13

In exercises done lying down on your side, you can flex the knee of the supporting leg in order to increase balance.

– This adaptation should only be used in cases when poor balance results in inadequate exercise technique for example in the side leg series.

Scoliosis

14. Arc behind back, no. 3

Resting the back on an arch eliminates any possible strain that might be caused by curvature of the spine.

–This adaptation can be used in exercises in which the trunk must be kept flexed, such as the hundred. It is also used in exercises where the trunk rolls backwards when you do not want the student to flop back completely, and in all the abdominal variations for the upper and lower body, placing the support a little closer to your neck and with your hands behind it.

15. Articulating the spine sitting down, no. 8

This adaptation should be used when you cannot roll on your back because of insufficient articular flexibility in the spine. In these cases, the spinal joints should be worked in less aggressive positions, eliminating any impact against the floor.

– This modification can be done instead of rolling on your back in the exercise Rolling Like a Ball.

16. Arc under the hips and lower back, no. 9

When back and abdominal muscles are not strong enough to keep your body weight in the air, you will need to compensate by placing a support under your lower back.

– This modification will enable you to do exercises such as "bicycling in air", which otherwise be more likely to cause injury than produce benefits.

17. Arc under hips and lower back with one supporting leg, no. 17/18

An arc will support your lower back and avoid strain if you suffer from lumbar scoliosis and in exercises that require you to support yourself with one or both feet on the floor while your trunk is raised.

– This adaptation can be used in the Bridge and any of its variations.

18. Hands on forehead, no. 21

Recommended in cases of dorsal scoliosis with pronounced kyphotic curve, even if it is only visible on one side of the back, and if poor mobility or adhesions make it uncomfortable and painful for you to put your hands behind your head.

— This adaptation can be used in every exercise in which you would normally place your hands behind your head. However, must take care not to hunch your back while doing the exercise.

19. Kneeling, no. 23

Some people suffering from scoliosis may find it difficult to lie face down and stretch their arms forwards, resulting in pain and potentially in injury. Any exercise demanding elevation is therefore inadvisable in the case of pathologies of this kind.

— Kneeling eliminates most of the workload in the exercises in which this modification can be used, but in a limited range of movements, it will enable scapular mobilization and produce benefits. For example, it can be used in the Swimming and similar exercises.

20. Flexed elbows, no. 24

Some people suffering from scoliosis may find it difficult to lie face down and stretch their arms forwards, resulting in pain and potentially in injury. Any exercise demanding elevation is therefore inadvisable in the case of pathologies of this kind. However, it is usually enough to flex your elbows and open your arms a little to change the work angle of the shoulders. This modification can be used in the Swimming and similar exercises.

21. Flexing the knees in the prone plank position, no. 26

You can reduce the intensity of leg pulls by flexing your knees, which will shorten the lever and reduce the effort for your back. It will also avoid pain in the knees caused by locking the knee joints.

— This modification will also make exercises like the front leg pull and the final part of the push-up easier.

22. One flexed knee in supine plank position, no. 27

If you lack sufficient strength or suffer from any back condition, you can reduce the size of the lever. In the original exercise, with outstretched knees, the gap between the supports provided by the hands and feet may be too long. You can vary the intensity of the exercise by changing the flexion of the knee: the more flexion, the less intensity.

— The exercise for which this adaptation is most clearly appropriate is the leg pull, though it can also be used in others that involve a similar position, including those done lying on your side with your legs or body elevated, like the side bend.

Shoulders

23. Cushion under the head while lying on your side, no. 11

If you feel discomfort or strain in the upper fibers of the trapezius, the upper deltoid or the rotators, you should avoid the compression that comes from resting your head on your arm.

— You can use a cushion whenever necessary in all exercises done lying on your side.

24. Cushion under the head while lying on your side with one arm forward, no. 12/28

Sometimes it is not enough to increase the space between your arm and your head to eliminate compression and you may need to remove the arm that is beneath you. In these cases you can pillow your head on a cushion of an appropriate height, which will depend on the size of your shoulders.

—You can use a cushion like this whenever necessary in all exercises done lying on your side.

25. Hands on forehead, no. 21

This modification is recommended in if you suffer from significant kyphosis, causing hypomobility of the shoulder girdle and where poor mobility and adhesions make it uncomfortable or painful to put your hands behind your head.

— This variation can be done in any exercise in which you would normally place your hands behind your head. Be careful to avoid hunching your back further, however.

26. Kneeling, no. 23

Lying face down and extending your arms forwards may cause pain in injured or stiff shoulders. If, the exercise demands elevation in addition to this stretch, some people may not be able to do it at all. Kneeling allows scapular mobilization and provides the attendant benefits, even though it will partially reduce the workload involved in the exercise.

— This modification can be used in the Swimming exercise and similar exercises.

27. Flexed Elbows, no. 24

Some people suffering shoulder injuries or stiffness in the scapular girdle may experience discomfort lying face down and stretching their arms forwards. Any exercise demanding elevation is therefore inadvisable in these cases. However, it is usually enough to flex your elbows and open your arms a little to change the work angle of the shoulders.

—This modification can be used in the Swimming and similar exercises.

Breathing difficulties/ Prominent nose

28. Cushion beneath forehead, no. 22

Putting your face too close to the floor can sometimes feel claustrophobic. The position may also feel uncomfortable if your nose presses against the mat. In these cases you can attain an anatomically reasonable distance by placing a cushion under your forehead.

— This support can be used in any exercise done lying face down, even though you place your hands in the right position that in this case would be on either side of your head.

29. Adapted breathing pattern, no. 10

Breathing exercises are important in themselves, since their goal being to increase respiratory efficiency. If you are doing abdominal work and you find that it interferes with your breathing, you should prioritize the respiratory goal and you complete the exercise sitting down.

— This is the perfect adaptation for the hundred, swapping the boat position for a sitting hundred.

Lower Back

30. Cushion under the hips in the prone lying position, no. 2

Using a cushion will avoid lower back pain in exercises done facing downwards. Resting your abdomen on a large, relatively soft surface will limit the extension of your lower back, allowing you to do exercises that would otherwise only cause further pain. Using a cushion is more moderate than using an arch and it is therefore recommended as an alternative to prevent lower back pain.

— This adaptation can be used in exercises like dorsal extension, heel squeeze prone, prone glute, one-leg kick and so on

31. Arc behind back, no. 3.

Resting your back against an arc eliminates most of your abdominal workload. Therefore, if you suffer lower back pain caused by lack of muscle tone, the arc will allay the strain felt in the lower back.

— An arc can also be used in exercises in which the trunk must be kept flexed, such as the hundred, and where the trunk is rolls backwards if you do not want the student to flop down completely. It is also suitable in all the abdominal variations for the upper and lower body, provided you place the support a little nearer to your neck and put your hands behind it.

32. Resistance Band under the Feet, no. 4

This adaptation reduces the effort required to counteract against gravity, which makes it appropriate to lessen the work of the lower back and ensure proper positioning of the neck.

— The resistance band can be used in half roll back and roll-up exercises, exercises involving elevation of the legs, and so forth, since it will protect your back if your abdomen is not yet strong enough to handle the workload. It is also appropriate for the menstrual period, certain stages of pregnancy, and in cases of chronic lower back pain or problems with the spinal discs.

33. Cushion under the hips in the supine position, no. 6

A cushion can be used to eliminate tension in the lower back due to tight muscles in the posterior chain or abdominal weakness.

— It is helpful in exercises like two-leg circles and corkscrews, where the student is lying on their back and the position of the legs produces an excessive curvature of the lower back.

34. Sitting on a cushion, no. 7

A cushion can be used to make sitting more comfortable if you suffer from title muscles in the posterior chain, especially the hamstring and glutes regions, and in the upper and lower back, which cause back pain.

— The cushion is used when it is impossible to keep the spine elongated during upper-body exercises done with small devices (pectoral press with ring, sitting hundred, articular mobilizations of the shoulders, stretches of the neck muscles, and so on).

35. Arc under the trunk in supine lying position, no. 5

Beginning with a stretch of the iliopsoas will reduce any strain the lower back in exercises that require extension of the hips.

— It is recommended that you stretch before these exercises, which are generally done lying prone like the prone glute, leg pull front and swimming.

36. Arc beneath trunk lying prone, number 13

An arc will help avoid lower back pain in exercises done face down. By supporting the abdomen on a rounded surface, the lower back also rounds effortlessly, allowing you to do exercises that would otherwise only cause further pain. The use of an arc is more conservative than that of a cushion and is recommended to allow people suffering from acute lower back pain to exercise.

— The adaptation can be used in exercises like dorsal extension, heel squeeze, prone glute and one-leg kick.

37. Raised foot support, no. 16

The extra work required of the hamstring muscles when you place your feet on a support, avoids excess in raising the trunk if closure of the ribcage has not been fully integrated.

— This adaptation can be used in the bridge and similar exercises. It will help relax the ribcage, making the sternum descend and accompanying the gesture with a deep exhalation.

38. Arc under the hips and lower back with one supporting leg, no. 17

The arc will support the lower back and avoid excessive curvature of the lower back (hyperlordosis) in exercises that involve supporting the feet on the floor while keeping your trunk in the air.

— It can be used in the bridge exercise or any of its variations.

39. Flexed knees, number 20

Sometimes no accessories are needed to make it easier to raise your legs without risk for your lower back, or to extend your legs in sitting exercises- All you need is to flex your knees to shorten the lever, reducing the effort needed to counteract gravity and the stretch in the muscle chains.

— You can do this in any exercise when you cannot extend your knees without injury or you find spinal elongation impossible.

40. Flexed knees in prone plank position, no. 26

You can reduce the intensity of leg pulls by flexing your knees, which will shorten the lever and reduce the effort for your back, as well as preventing knee pain caused by locking the knee joint.

— This modification makes exercises like the leg pull front, final part of the push-up and so on easier.

Wrists

41. Supine forearm support, no. 25

You can this modification to avoid supporting your weight on your wrists if you suffer from chronic or acute pain. However, it requires more attention to scapular stabilization, to prevent the common mistake of hunching your shoulders up to your ears when the gap between your head and the floor is reduced.

— The modification is helpful in both prone and supine front leg pull exercises, in mixed abdominals on hand support and in exercises that work the abdominal transverse with diagonally raised legs. It can also be used in the side bend and its lateral abdominals variation.

42. Prone forearm support, no. 28

This modification eliminates the need to support your weight on your the wrists in case of chronic or acute pain. This variation requires more attention to scapular stabilization, however, because of the common hunching your shoulders up by your ears when the gap between your head and the floor is reduced.

— This adaptation is suitable for the front prone and supine leg pull exercises, mixed abdominals on hand support and in exercises that work the abdominal transverse with diagonally raised legs. It can also used in the side bend and its variation for lateral abdominals.

Knees

43. Cushion under the knees lying prone, number 19

If you suffer from soft knee cartilage, flexion of the joints in the prone lying position can cause pain due to the contact of your kneecap with the floor and your femur. Use a cushion to isolate your knee from the floor and provide a soft point of contact.

— Used in exercises like the one-leg kick and similar.

44. Mat under knees in the kneeling position, no. 14

Flexing your knees deeply can cause pain for people suffering cartilage conditions. In this case, you need to increase the angle of flexion by placing a rolled-up mat, a cushion or a blanket in the hollow of the knees.

— This adaptation can be used in the shell stretch and similar exercises.

45. Flexed knees in the prone plank position, no. 26

You can reduce the intensity of leg pulls by flexing your knees, which will shorten the lever and reduce the effort for your back. It will also prevent pain caused by locking the knee joints.

— This adaptation will make exercises like the front leg pull and the final part of the push-up easier.

46. One flexed knee in supine plank position, no. 27

If the knees are slack and form the middle of the support lever it is recommended not to reach lock out the joints. You can do this by flexing them, which will make the exercise will be more or less intense the more flexion, the less intensity.

— This adaptation is clearly recommended is the leg pull. However, it can also be used in any exercise requiring a similar posture, including those done from the side with the body elevated, like the side bend.

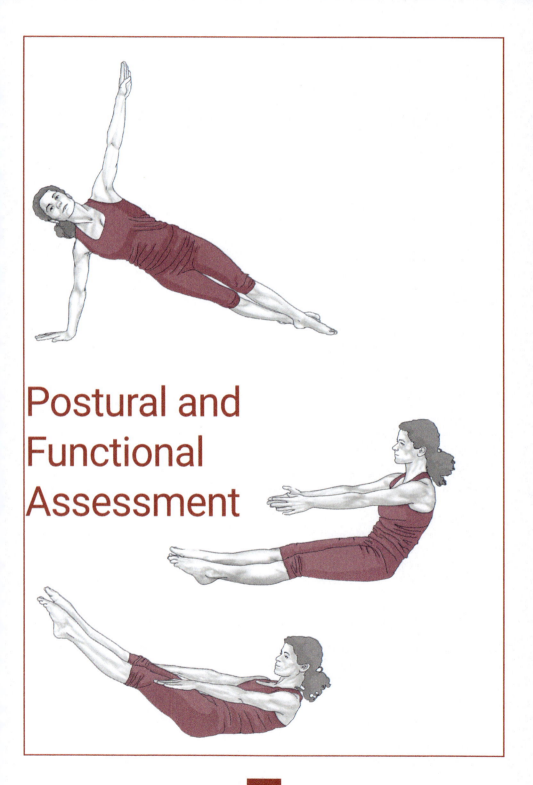

Postural and Functional Assessment

Postural Assessment

Why is postural assessment necessary?

Being aware of our own or, in the case of professionals, of our students' posture is essential to establish a basis on which to design a training routine. Poor bodily alignment stresses the musculoskeletal system.

Postural and functional assessment provides the clues needed to set both health, aesthetic and fitness goals.

Everything is connected. Working to improve your posture and postural habits is the best way to improve your physical appearance, while the pursuit of enhanced fitness in a context of health and progress achieved through will help you achieve a better proportioned, leaner, stronger, nimbler, more dynamic and more youthful physique.

Hasty assessments of a person's physical condition and structure can often lead to false conclusions, and this means that time must be taken to make a methodical study of each individual's different body segments and their peculiarities. For instance, a person may appear at first glance to suffer from hyperlordosis or hollow back syndrome when actually he or she merely has prominent glutes. Hence you need to observe the position of the hips (the anterior superior iliac spines in relation to the groin) to be certain of the supposed condition, otherwise you will take the wrong approach to your work with the student in question.

It is also important to tell poor posture resulting from bad habits apart structural problems. Habits can be changed in order to correct posture, but it is far from easy to modify a person's physical structure, and in most cases you should not even try. The key in such cases is to balance the whole while respecting the structure.

Observing your posture in a mirror from the front, side and back (in this case you will have to seek help, because you must not only look but also maintain a natural standing position). Avoid any temptation to color what you are seeing, but stay objective and impartial. Simply jot down any deviations you may observe according to the following outline. You may also need to touch some body parts to confirm what your eyes are telling you. Let us do it.

Front View

	Head				
Centered	Tilted to the right	Tilted to the left	Turned to the right	Turned to the left	Other

	Shoulders				
Aligned	Right shoul-der lower	Left shoulder higher	Inward rota-tion	Outward rotation	Other

	Ribcage				
Aligned	Rotation to right	Rotation to left	Low		Other

	Pelvis				
Crests aligned	Right low	Left high			Other

	Knees				
Aligned	Valgus	Varus			Other

	Ankles				
Aligned	Valgus	Varus			Other

	Feet				
Normal	Flat	Hollow	Pronated	Supinated	Other

Head

Centered: Same distance from right and left ears to right and left shoulders, respectively.

Tilted: One ear is tilted towards the shoulder, while the other is tilted away.

Turned: Sideways displacement of the head out of the vertical axis ("Egyptians head").

Shoulders

Aligned: Both shoulders at the same height, forming a horizontal axis parallel to the floor.

Low: One shoulder below the level of the horizontal axis and downward pointing collarbone.

High: One shoulder below the level of the horizontal axis and upward pointing collarbone.

Rotated: An easy way to observe inward or outward rotation of the shoulders is the pen test. Hold two pens in your fists, one in each hand, and let your arms drop slack to your sides. If the points of the pens point inwards, there is internal rotation; if they point outwards, there is external rotation.

Ribcage

Aligned: Ribs at the same height on both sides, forming a horizontal axis.

Rotation: Internal edge of the ribs approaching the central axis.

Low: One side of the ribcage is lower.

High: One side of the ribcage is higher.

Pelvis

Aligned: Both iliac crests at the same height.

High or low: High or low crest in relation to the fourth lumbar vertebra (L4).

Knees

Aligned: Kneecaps with anterior side looking forwards, without lateral displacement.

Valgus: Knock-knees so that the legs form an X-shape with lateral flexion towards the medial plane.

Varus: Bow legs, so that the legs form parentheses ( ) with the knees flexed towards the lateral plane.

Ankles

Aligned: Continuing the verticality of the tibia towards the floor.

Valgus: Flexion towards the medial plane so that the toes are pointing inward.

Varus: Flexion towards the lateral plane so that the toes are pointing outward.

Feet

Normal: Body weight distributed between toes, heel and external lateral and medial of the foot sole.

Flat: Body weight on the entire sole, with main support on the inside of the foot.

Hollow: Body weight on the outside of the foot.

Pronator: Valgus ankle and tendency to flat foot.

Supinator: Varus ankle and tendency to hollow foot. Vista lateral

Vista lateral

Head				
Centered	Tilted	Tilted bac-		Other

Cervical Vertebrae (Neck)				
Normal curve	Hyperlordosis	Flat		Other

Thoracic or Dorsal Vertebrae (Upper back)				
Normal Curve	Hyperkypho-	Flat	Military	Other

Lumbar Vertebrae (Lower back)				
Normal Curve	Hyperlordosis	Hyperkypho-		Other

Pelvis				
Neutral	Anteversion	Retroversion		Other

Knees				
Normal flexion	Hyperexten-	Hyperflexion		Other

Ankles				
Normal flexion	Dorsal flexion	Plantar flexion		Other

Head

Centered: The vertical axis passes through the crown of the head, running down through the earlobe, the ear canal and the odontoid apophysis of the axis vertebra.

Tilted forwards: The vertical axis passes behind the earlobe.

Tilted backwards: The vertical axis passes in front of the earlobe.

Cervical Vertebrae (Neck)

Normal curve: The vertical axis passes straight through the cervical vertebrae.

Hyperlordosis: Increased cervical lordosis. The vertical axis passes behind the cervical vertebrae. Excessively curved neck.

Flat: Rectification of cervical hyperlordosis. Neck without curve.

Thoracic or Dorsal Vertebrae (Upper back)

Normal curve: Slightly convex backwards curve in relation to the vertical axis.

Hyperkyphosis: Increased dorsal kyphosis or hunched back. Very pronounced backwards curve.

Flat: Flat upper back. Rectification of dorsal kyphosis. No backward curve in relation to the vertical axis.

Military: Raised and puffed-out thorax. Rectification of dorsal kyphosis

Lumbar Vertebrae (Lower back)

Normal Curve: Slightly convex forward curve in relation to the vertical axis.

Hyperlordosis: Exaggerated forward curve in the lower back in relation to the vertical axis accompanied by forward pelvic tilt (commonly known as "swayback")

Hyperkyphosis: Reduced curve in the lower back, accompanied by backward pelvic tilt (rounded hips).

Pelvis

Neutral: The anterior superior iliac spines coincide in a vertical plane, perpendicular to the floor, with the pubic symphysis.

Anteversion: The anterior superior iliac spines are in front of the vertical plane.

Retroversion: The anterior superior iliac spines are behind the vertical plane.

Knees

Normal flexion: The vertical axis runs slightly in front of the center of the knee joint.

Hyperflexion: Forward knees forwards. Usually associated with dorsal flexion of the ankles.

Hyperextension: Backward knees. Usually associated plantar flexion of the ankles.

Ankles

Normal flexion: Vertical tibia at a 90-degree angle to the sole of the foot.

Dorsal flexion: More flexion towards the back of the foot. The ankle appears flexed.

Plantar flexion: More flexion towards the sole of the foot. The ankle appears more extended.

Back View

Shoulder Blades				
Normal	Winged	Frozen		Other

Spine				
Aligned	Scoliosis	Discontinuity		Other

Pelvis				
Normal PSIS	Excessive	Defective PSIS		Other

ASIS: anterior superior iliac spines. **PSIS:** posterior superior iliac spines.

Shoulder Blades

Normal: Feel the edge of the shoulder blade in the neutral (anatomical) position. You should just be able to insert the tip of your finger between the shoulder blade and your ribs.

Winged: The shoulder blades protrude away from the medial part of the ribcage (near the spine). You can insert the first phalanx of your finger.

Frozen: You cannot insert your fingers and can barely feel the edges of the shoulder blades.

Spine

Aligned: Straight, without deviating from the vertical axis.

Scoliosis: With curves. Simple or double scoliosis.

Pelvis

Normal anterior superior iliac spines: Two tiny hollows of about the same size a fingertip can be seen on either side of the sacrum.

Excessive anterior superior iliac spines: The hollows are enlarged.

Defective anterior superior iliac spines: The hollows are not visible.

Articulation

Spine, Front Flexion				
Continuity	Flat			Other

Spine, Lateral Flexion				
Normal Flexion	Discontinuity			Other

Shoulder Blades

Normal: Feel the edge of the shoulder blade in the neutral (anatomical) position. You should just be able to insert the tip of your finger between the shoulder blade and your ribs.

Winged: The shoulder blades protrude away from the medial part of the ribcage (near the spine). You can insert the first phalanx of your finger.

Frozen: You cannot insert your fingers and can barely feel the edges of the shoulder blades.

Spine

Aligned: Straight, without deviating from the vertical axis.

Scoliosis: With curves. Simple or double scoliosis.

Pelvis

Normal anterior superior iliac spines: Two tiny hollows of about the same size a fingertip can be seen on either side of the sacrum.

Excessive anterior superior iliac spines: The hollows are enlarged.

Defective anterior superior iliac spines: The hollows are not visible.

Pen Test

Shoulder Rotation				
No rotation	Inward right	Outward left	Inward right	Outward left

This test easily measures inward or outward shoulder rotation. Hold two pens in your fists, one in each hand, and let your arms drop slack to your sides. Now observe whether the points of the pens turn inwards (internal rotation) or outwards (external rotation). Inward rotations is associated with overload in the front and outward rotation with overload in the back of your shoulders.

Functional Assessment

As soon as we begin to move we start to pick up bad postural habits, which have negative effects on our physical wellbeing. Imagine a baby trying day after day to suck the big toe on her right foot. The muscles on that side of her hips will be more elongated at the back than on the left side but shorter in front. It may not be obvious, but the baby's musculoskeletal system is already becoming imbalanced.

Now transfer this image to your own everyday life and put yourself in our baby's place. How many pernicious movements do you repeat throughout your day? Which of the postures you adopt disrupt your muscular balance? Do your joints move according to the right biomechanical patterns? Do you generate more physical strain than necessary? Are you aware of poor posture, or do you only realize when you begin to feel pain?

Functional assessment provides data on these imbalances at both the articular and the muscular level. It will reveal if one side of our bodies has become stronger than the other. It will help you assess the strength of your different muscle groups and understand, in view of your everyday activities and exercise habits, why some muscle groups are strong but others are weak, and why some joints conserve their full range of movement but others have become stiff, some of them so much so as to affect your quality of life and personal autonomy.

It is important to counteract these imbalances, and the best way to do this is to know them? A few simple exercises will provide a general idea of your own or a student's condition. Some of these exercises are part of the Pilates method and others are drawn from the world of fitness but can be performed applying Pilates principles of the Method to increase the scope of the assessment.

How to assess and determine level in the Pilates method

Each exercise has its own function within the assessment, touching on different issues. The sum of all the parts is what provide you with an all round view of your own or a student's level, while analysis of each exercise will focus the training design.

For instance, if a practitioner scores 3 on the half squat exercise but 2 on the full squat exercise because their heels come up off the floor, training should be oriented more towards stretching the calf muscles than strengthening the quadriceps. However, only one repetition is not enough to gauge the actual strength of the practitioner's quadriceps, but only to establish that the base is good. In contrast, the base in terms of the calf stretch is not good. Following up with the balance en relevé (tiptoes balance) exercise, you will find out if the calf muscles are strong, while with the quadriceps stretch will show if the muscles are elastic.

The assessment process can be complex, then, but this complexity is part and parcel of taking charge of your own or someone else's training.

Scoring

Even though the tables are based on a range of scores from 0 to 3, fractions can also be used to hone the assessment. This option will depend on the demands imposed for successful completion of an exercise. If you decide to use fractional scores, you will need to establish a scorecard, a personal assessment that is always applied in the same situations. Assessing function is complicated because there are lots of variations on what the ideal execution of a given exercise actually consists of. The scores proposed here are a valid example to obtain data on your own or a student's functionality, but any assessment is valid as long as it offers the user full information on movement range, strength, shortenings and articular mobility.

What if I can't do an exercise at all?

It doesn't matter. The exercise scores zero and you continue with the others. The most important thing is to learn the reason why you cannot do it. Is it because of an injury? Is it because the practitioner is not strong enough? Or not flexible enough? Information exchange is necessary because what we see is rarely the whole story, and if we do not ask we risk drawing false conclusions.

Exercises

Strength assessment

Half Squat

This exercise assesses mainly the strength of quadriceps, tibialis anterior, and spinal elongation with flexion of the hips.

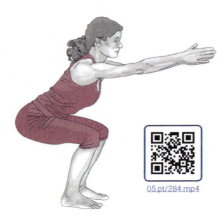

05.pt/284.mp4

Flex your knees 90 degrees while leaning your trunk forwards.

3 points: knees flexed 90 degrees, neutral hips, trunk leaning forwards and spine elongated.

2 points: knees flexed 90 degrees, hips in retroversion, trunk leaning forwards and spine not elongated.

1 point: knees too far forward and flexed over 90 degrees, hips in retroversion, trunk leaning forwards and spine not elongated.

Full Squat

This exercise assesses mainly the strength of the quadriceps and tibialis anterior, the elasticity of the calf muscles and the elongation of the spine with flexion of the hips.

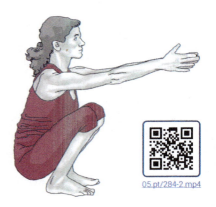

05.pt/284-2.mp4

Flex your knees completely until the backs of your thighs meet your calves.

3 points: Deep flexion of the knees until the thighs meet the calves with the heels flat on the floor, hips in slight retroversion and spine elongated.

2 points: Deep flexion of the knees, with the heels not flat on the floor, hips in slight retroversion and the spine not elongated.

1 point: Limited flexion of the knees, heels not flat on the floor, hips in wide retroversion and spine not elongated.

Standing Balance Relevé

This exercise assesses mainly balance and the strength of the calf muscles.

Triceps Push-up

This exercise assesses mainly the strength of the pectorals, serrates and abdomen.

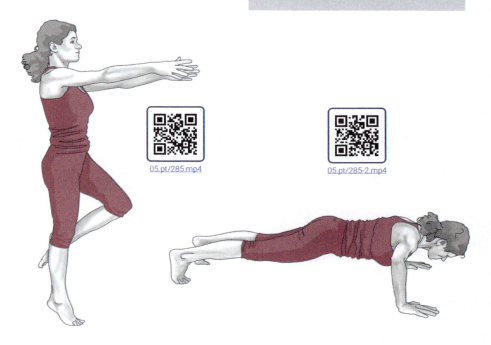

05.pt/285.mp4

05.pt/285-2.mp4

Three elevations standing on one foot on tiptoes, keeping the other leg flexed and its foot at calf height.

3 points: Three complete elevations per foot with total balance and fluidity.

2 points: Three complete elevations per foot.

1 point: Unable to do three elevations.

Start from the prone plank position with your arms shoulder-width apart, your elbows flexed and your hands in line with your chest.

3 points: Complete elevation of the trunk in prone plank position.

2 points: Complete elevation of the trunk without maintaining the plank.

1 point: Difficulty elevating the trunk and imbalance between the right and left sides of the body.

Lateral Elevation

This exercise assesses mainly the strength of abdominal obliques and serrates.

Superman 1

This exercise assesses mainly the strength of the glutes, lower back and medial dorsal muscles.

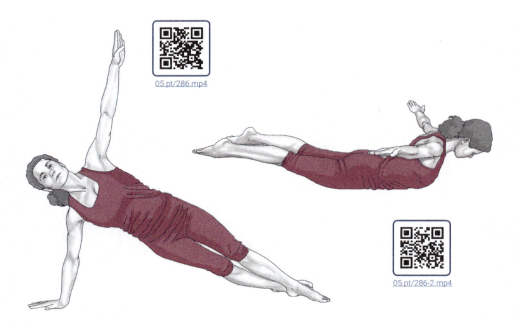

05.pt/286.mp4

05.pt/286-2.mp4

Do the second position of the Side Bend (exercise 13, level 2, Mixed)

3 points: Elevation of the trunk maintaining good balance in the frontal plane, without rotation.

2 points: Elevation of the trunk maintaining balance with difficulty and with some rotation.

1 point: Need to modify the support of feet or hands to raise the trunk.

From a prone lying position, raise your trunk, head and legs with your arms spread out to form a cross.

3 points: Well-proportioned elevation of trunk, head and legs while maintaining axial elongation.

2 points: Upper body elevated above the level of the lower body, or vice versa, and loss of axial elongation.

1 point: Elevation of one half of the body only.

Superman 2

This exercise assesses mainly the strength of the posterior deltoid and the medial dorsal muscles.

Hundred

This exercise assesses mainly the strength of the abdominal muscles.

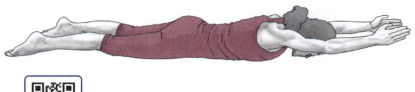

05.pt/287.mp4

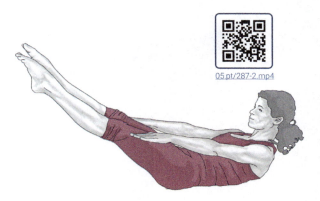

05.pt/287-2.mp4

Lying prone with your forehead resting on the floor, raise your arms forwards.

3 points: Arms raised with extended elbows.

2 points: Arms raised with flexed elbows.

1 point: Only one arm raised.1 punto.

Flex your trunk and raise your lower body, with your arms stretched forwards.

3 points: Hold for 30 seconds maintaining good posture.

2 points: Hold for 30 seconds with modified posture.

1 point: Able to achieve the right posture but not to hold it for 30 seconds.

Raised Leg with Knee Support

Valora, principalmente, la fuerza de los abductores de la cadera.

To Value Range of Movement

Roll-Up

This exercise assesses mainly the articular flexibility of the spine in flexion and abdominal strength.

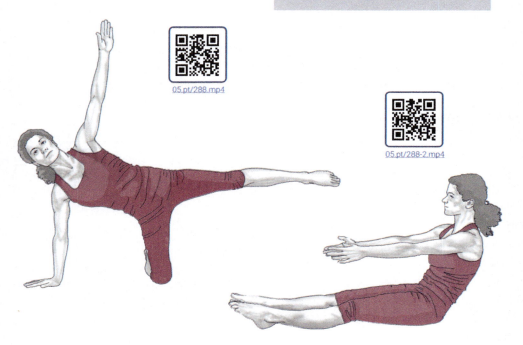

05.pt/288.mp4

05.pt/288-2.mp4

Lying on one side, supported on one hand and knee. Raise one leg up to hip height, keeping your trunk and legs aligned in the frontal plane without rotation.

3 points: Hold for 30 seconds with good posture.

2 points: Hold out for 30 seconds with modified posture but keeping the leg raised.

1 point: Able to achieve the right posture but not to hold it for 30 seconds with the leg raised.

Sitting down, extend your trunk vertebra by vertebra until you are lying on your back, then return to the starting position, again vertebra by vertebra.

3 points: Complete elevation, fluid, harmonious and steady.

2 points: Complete elevation, jerky movement in spurts.

1 point: Cannot lower or raise the trunk properly.

Post

This exercise assesses mainly the functionality of the shoulders.

05.pt/289.mp4

Cobra

This exercise assesses mainly the flexibility of the spine in extension.

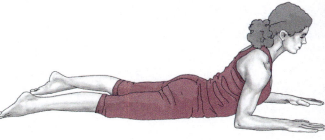

05.pt/289-2.mp4

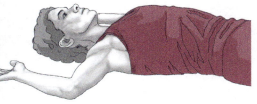

With heels, hips, back and skull flat against a wall, raise your arms from a 90-degree flexion of the elbows.

3 points: 20-centimeter elevation with the whole forearm flat against the wall.

2 points: 20-centimeter elevation with only elbows or hands flat against the wall.

1 point: Elevation of the arms but inability to keep them flat against the wall.

Lying prone, extend your spine while supporting your forearms on the floor.

3 points: The hips stay flat on the floor, the shoulders are retracted away from ears and the arms stay glued to the sides.

2 points: The hips stay flat on the floor and/or the shoulders hunch forward towards the ears and the arms stay glued to the sides.

1 point: Cannot achieve forearm support without detaching the arms from the sides.

Sitting Down

This exercise assesses mainly the elasticity of the posterior chain of the lower body, as well as spinal elongation.

Sitting Down with Legs Open

This exercise assesses mainly the elasticity of the posterior chain of the upper body, as well as the flexibility of the adductors.

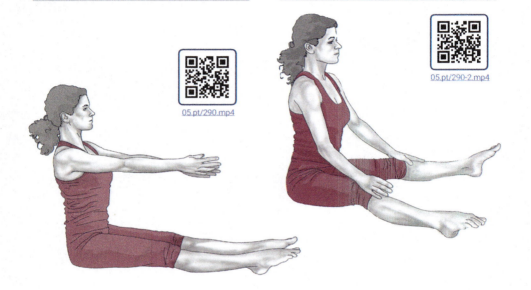

05.pt/290.mp4

05.pt/290-2.mp4

Sit with legs hip-width apart and knees extended.

3 points: Spine elongated, hips neutral, knees extended.

2 points: Spine flexed, hips neutral, knees extended.

1 point: Spine flexed, hips in retroversion, knees flexed.

Sit with legs one meter apart about wide and knees extended.

3 points: Spine elongated, hips neutral, knees extended.

2 points: Spine flexed, hips neutral, knees extended.

1 point: Spine flexed, hips in retroversion, knees flexed.

Z-Sit

This exercise assesses mainly the internal and external hip rotators.

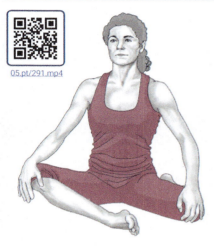

05.pt/291.mp4

Sit with legs positioned like a letter Z.

3 points: Both ischia rest on the floor, spine elongated.

2 points: One ischium only on the floor, spine elongated.

1 point: One ischium only on the floor, spine not elongated.

Quadriceps Stretch

This exercise assesses mainly the elasticity of the quadriceps and iliopsoas.

05.pt/291-2.mp4

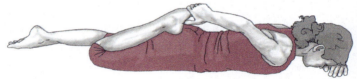

Lying prone, flex one knee and pull the heel to the glute with the aid of the hand.

3 points: Heel touches glute, hips stay extended and spine stays elongated.

2 points: Heel touches glute and spine stays elongated, but the hips flex.

1 point: Heel hardly approaches glute, hips flex and spine loses elongation.

Preparation of an Anatomical and Functional Assessment Report

The first step is to prepare a background report by completing a questionnaire regarding aspects of the subject's everyday life, medical history and current situation in terms of pain, illness and activity.

Questionnaire	
Date:	
Name:	
Age:	
Job and Workplace Posture:	Shopworker. Standing and sitting down. Carrying light loads.
Initial Goals	Improve agility, flexibility and core physical fitness. Im- prove abdominal tone and achieve weight loss. Leisure
Sports	No sports background. Occasional fitness workouts
Medical History	An old sprain in the right knee causes pain with exercise. Inflammation (CMP) of the right knee. Dorsal scoliosis to the right.
Recurring Pain	Right knee and cervical overload.
Surgery	None

Postural Assessment	
Front View	Valgus ankles, more on the right than the left, valgus knees, left shoulder raised and head tilted to the right
Lateral View	Slight cervical kyphosis, shoulders thrust forwards, ges- tural advance of the head to compensate for cervical kyphosis, slack joints
Posterior View	Dorsal scoliosis to the right.
Spinal Flexion	More development of the muscles on the right side, poor articulation of the lower back

Functional Assessment

Score: 1.82 out of 3.

Score is obtained by adding up the scores of all the exercises assessed, then dividing the result by the quantity of exercises.

Half squat	Not finished due to shortening of calf muscles
Full squat	Head tilted forward with neck pain due to shortening of poste- rior chain
Balance en relevé	Better on the left foot due to right-footedness/dextrality
Triceps push-up	Arched back due to lack of abdominal tone
Lateral leg elevation	Impossible due to insufficient support on the left knee caused by lateral abdominal weakness. Right side complete, with knee pain due to articular instability
Superman	Right side weaker in glute and back
Prone arms elevation	Left side weak
Hundred	Good
Raised leg with knee support	Cannot position the trunk in the frontal plane. Poor lateral flexibility
Roll-up	Complete, but with poor dorso-lumbar articulation
Post	Difficulty and effort
Cobra	Poor articulation
Sitting down neutral	Shortened posterior chain
Sitting down with open legs	Shortening of adductors and posterior chain, though less
Z-sit (right)	Pain in the knee (internal lateral ligament or meniscus), right hip raised, spine not elongated
Sitting like a Z (left)	No pain in the knee and better placement of hips and spine
Prone knee flexion	Correct
Pen test (see "Postural assessment" tests)	Internal rotation of both shoulders.

Goals

1. Elongation work on the posterior muscle chain
2. Elongation work on the calf muscles
3. Work to improve muscular balance between left and right sides
4. Work on upper body bilaterality for scoliosis management
5. Work to strengthen the shallow and deep layers of the abdomen
6. Work to strengthen the thigh muscles for stability of the right knee
7. Work on lumbodorsal articulation
8. Work to strengthen f the medial dorsal muscles (between the shoulder blades)
9. Adductor flexibility work
10. Flexibility work on the external rotators of the right hip

After completing the assessment report, it is to review to review the resulting goals and make a table or list of exercises with which to work on the target areas identified. In the example case, this would involve using the Cat and Horse, Saw and similar exercises to work on elongation of the posterior chain.

Elongation or elasticity of the calf muscles can be achieved using any exercise that requires flexo-extension of the ankles or even including work to stretch the hamstrings and calves (p. 192).

The achievement of muscular balance between both sides of the body requires meticulous attention while you are the exercises to ensure that you do the movements in exactly the same way on one side and then the other, however difficult this may seem and even if you do not at first succeed fully. In addition to your own conscious awareness, mirror can be a helpful aid for this purpose.

Bilaterality work on the upper body for scoliosis management means that you should be careful to prevent your arms, shoulder blades and spine from drifting back into the more comfortable position allowed by the scoliotic curve. For example, when you do the Swimming exercise (p.130), try to raise both arms to the same height. You will of course have more difficulty on one side if you suffer from scoliosis, but you should avoid overworking the other arm (i.e. raise it only as far as the weaker arm other will go). This is the key to achieving bilateral balance. Naturally, I take for granted that you will put maximum effort into raising the weaker arm. All of the exercises that alternate the work between the two sides of your body are ideal to help scoliosis sufferers maintain a healthy.

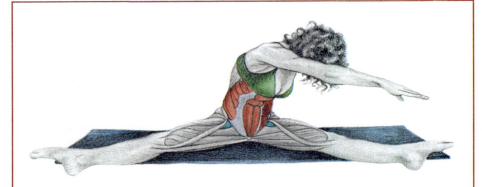

Annexes

To strengthen the shallow and deep layers of the abdomen, you will need to focus on the abdominal exercises dealt with in a category of their own in this book. The exercises must be done properly according to the Principles of the Method, otherwise you will not engage the deep layers and your abdomen will take on the characteristic bumpy form visible when the deep fibers are unattended, and your abdomen will fail to perform its key function as protector of the back.

Using the above method, you will be able to create a list of exercises appropriate to the person assessed. If you are using a previous assessment, you will already be working on particular goals, of course, and you can also jump right in without any assessment. This is fine, although your goals in such case you goals will necessarily be more general.

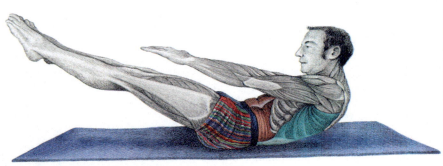

Even if your goals are general, however, Pilates is a very efficient way to keep your body fit and healthy. So come on, choose ten different exercises and start training!

Annex 1
Exercises by Level

Level 1

1-1.	Ab Prep	47
2-1	Breast Stroke	176
3-1	Hundred	50
4-1.	Half Roll Back	53
5-1	Roll Up	56
6-1	One Leg Circle	143
7-1	Twist	105
8-1	Rolling Like a Ball	58
9-1	One Leg Stretch	60
10-1	One Leg Stretch Oblique	62
11-1	Double Leg Stretch	64
12-1.	Scissors	67
13-1	Hell Squeeze Prone	145
14-1.	Saw	107
15-1.	Half Roll Back Obliques	69
16-1	One Leg Kick	147
17-1	Side Leg Series	150

18-1	Trunk and Legs Lateral Elevation	109
19-1	Axial Flexion	72
20-1	Single Leg Extensión	153
21-1.	seal	74
22-1	shell stretch	169
23-1	cat and horse	111
24-1	trunk rotation	76
25-1	supine squad	114
26-1	abdominal series	78
27-1	prone gluteo	155

Level 2

1-2	Slow Double Leg Stretch	81
2-2.	Bridge	157
3-2	Roll Over	84
4-2	One Leg Kick	160
5-2	Open Leg Rocker	86
6-2	Roll Up Advanced	88
7-2	Jackknife	91
8-2	Double Leg Kick	116
9-2	Teaser	93
10-2	Swimming	119
11-2	Leg Pull Front	121
12-2	Hip Twist	96
13-2	Side Bend	123
14-2	Push Up	126
15-2	Hinge	163

Level 3

1-3	Scissors in Air	129
2-3	Teaser Series	98
3-3	Swan Dive	132
4-3	Leg Pull	135
5-3	Control Balance	138
6-3	Corks Crew	100
7-3	Side Kick Kneeling	140
8-3	Rocking	165
9-3	Boomerang	102

Annex 2

Glossary

Abduction: Movement of a limb or any other part of the body away from the central line that divides the body into symmetric left and right halves. Abducting your legs is the same as opening them.

Adduction: Movement of a limb or any part of the other body towards the central middle line that divides the body into symmetric left and right halves. Adducting your legs is the same as closing them.

Antepulsion: Movement of the shoulders that consists raising the arm in the sagittal plane. Raising the arms forwards.

Anteversion: Movement of the hips that consists of moving the ischia backwards and at the same projecting the anterior superior iliac spines (ASIS) forwards.

Basal metabolic rate: Daily energy expenditure that the body needs to carry out vital functions and other activities.

Concentric Contraction: Process by which a muscle is tensed and shortened to overcome a resistance, so as to move a part of your body. An example would be a biceps curl, in which you lift a weight with your hand and flex your elbow to bring it up to your shoulder.

Dynamic muscles: Muscles that shorten or lengthen depending on the movement performed. Dynamic muscles work thanks by isotonic contraction (combination of concentric and eccentric contractions).

Eccentric Contraction: Process by which a muscle is tensed and lengthened to overcome a resistance, so as to move a part of your body. The segments involved in eccentric contraction move away from each other, for example the movement of your arm when you take a glass from your lips and place it on the table.

Economy of effort: Broad concept consisting of minimizing the expenditure of energy required for a given action.

Endurance: Capacity to maintain an act of strength for a given lapse of time. An individual's level of endurance is determined by training of energetic metabolism, muscle adaptations and the capacity of the neuromuscular system to resist nervous fatigue.

Flexibility: Ability to achieve a broad range of movement in different positions.

Functional reeducation: Learning and training of new or forgotten patterns of motion in order to improve one's health and fitness.

Genu valgum (knock knees): Inward curvature of the legs, so that when the knees are together the feet are forced apart in the anatomical position. This condition is much more common in women than in men. If acute, it is considered a pathology.

Genu varum (bow legs): Outward the legs, so that the knees are forced apart when the feet are together in the anatomical position. This condition is much more common in men than in women. If acute, it is considered a pathology.

Isometric Contraction: Process by which a muscle is tensed without movement, so that it is not shortened or lengthened. An example would be carrying a tray on one hand and transporting its weight without moving your elbow.

Kyphosis: Convex spinal curvature in the dorsal region.

Mobility: Component of flexibility consisting of the ability of the joints have to make certain kinds of movement, depending on their morphology.

Muscle elasticity: Capacity of the muscles to lengthen and shorten, and to return to their original shape when the action ceases.

Muscle strain: Repetitive strain on affecting the muscular-tendinous system, resulting in a risk of injury. Muscle strain can be avoiding tweaking the training program to take into account an individual's traits, strengths and weaknesses.

Muscle strength: Capacity of the muscles to produce maximum muscle tension. This is the expression of muscle strength transmitted to the bone by means of the tendon.

Postural muscles: Deep muscle groups that hold posture in movement and active repose. They are similar to the stabilizing muscles, but they use less energy smaller energy once a movement has become automatic as a result of training.

Postural reeducation: Learning or recall of good posture thanks to observation of one's own body and the application of necessary changes.

Proprioception: Sense that allows perception of the body's position and awareness of its relationship to space and movement.

Retroversion: Movement of the hips that consists of pushing the ischia forwards and projecting the anterior superior iliac spines (ASIS) backwards.

Scoliosis: Abnormal S-shaped or C-shaped curvature of the spine, visible from the frontal plane. It can be congenital (present since birth), idiopathic (unknown causes) or neuromuscular (secondary symptom of another condition).

Speed of movement: The process of completing a movement as quickly as possible. In Pilates, only advanced-level aerial exercises require speed of movement at any time.

Stabilizing muscles: Muscles that keep a part of the body motionless while some of its segments are in motion. Stabilizing muscles work by isometric contractions.

Annex 3
Bibliography

- Alter, M. J. Manual de estiramientos deportivos. 4ª edición. Edit. Tutor. 2003.

- American College of Sports Medicine. Manual de consulta para el control y la prescripción de ejercicio. Edit. Paidotribo. 2000.

- Calais-Germain, B. Anatomía para el movimiento. Tomo I. Análisis de las técnicas corporales. Edit. La Liebre de Marzo. 1994.

- Calais-Germain, B.; Lamotte, A. Anatomía para el movimiento. Bases de ejercicios. Tomo II. Edit. La Liebre de Marzo.

- Calais-Germain, B. El periné femenino y el parto. Anatomía para el movimiento 3. Edit. La Liebre de Marzo.

- Calais-Germain, B. La respiración. El gesto respiratorio. Anatomía para el movimiento. Edit. La Liebre de Marzo.

- Calderón, F. J. Fisiología aplicada al deporte. Edit. Tebar. 2001.

- Craze, R. La técnica Alexander. 2ª edición. Edit. Paidotribo. 2002.

- Egoscue, P.; Gittines, R. Pain free. A revolution method for stopping chronic pain. Edit. Bantam Books. 1998.

- Egoscue, P.; Gittines, R. Pain free for women. The revolutionary program for ending chronic pain. Edit. Bantam Books. 2003.

- Egoscue, P.; Gittines, R. The Egoscue method of health through motion. Edit. Quill. 1992.

- Goyton, M. D.; Hall, Ph. D. Tratado de fisiología médica. 9ª edición. Edit. McGraw-Hill Interamericana. 1996.

- Hage, M. El gran libro del dolor de espalda. Edit. Paidós. 2006.

- Kendall, F. P.; Kendall McKreary, E. Músculos. Pruebas y funciones. 2ª edición. Edit. Jims. 1985.

- López Chicharro, J., Fernández Vaquero, A. Fisiología del ejercicio. 2ª edición. Edit. Médica Panamericana. 1998.

- Luttgens, K.; Wells, K. F. Kinesiología. Bases científicas del movimiento humano. 7ª edición. 1985.

- Lyle, J.; Micheli, M. D.; Jenkins, M. La nueva medicina deportiva. Edit. Tutor. 1998.

- Moore, K. L. Anatomía con orientación clínica. 3ª edición. Edit. Médica Panamericana. 1993.

- Netler, M. D. Atlas de anatomía humana. 4ª edición. Edit. Elsevier Masson. 2007.

- Prentice, W. E. Técnicas de rehabilitación en la medicina deportiva. 2ª edición. Edit. Paidotribo. 1999.

- Sampayo, S. Estiramientos y conciencia corporal. Edit. Edad. 2008.

- Souchard, Ph. E. Stretching Global Activo I. De la perfección muscular a los resultados deportivos. 4ª edición. Edit. Paidotribo. 2003.

- Souchard, Ph. E. Stretching Global Activo II. 4ª edición. Edit. Paidotribo. 2006.

- Ylinen, J. Estiramientos terapéuticos en el deporte y en las terapias manuales. Edit. Elsevier Masson. 2009.

3rd edition, updated

Printed by Amazon Italia Logistica S.r.l.
Torrazza Piemonte (TO), Italy